ADDITIONAL PRAISE *FOR NOT MY BUDDY*

"*Not My Buddy* is about Tracey Berkowitz's journey recovering from a condition that continues to be misunderstood by conventional medicine. Sadly, her story is not an exception. There are many people struggling with serious digestive issues directly related to undiagnosed parasitic infections. If it weren't for Tracey's courage and determination to share her story, I, for one, would not have met Dr. Cahill, who diagnosed me correctly and helped put me on the road back to health."

— LOUISE VYENT, former "supermodel" and public relations consultant

"Tracey's account of her battle with chronic giardiasis chronicles not only the physical and emotional struggles such patients face, but the fear, confusion and strain it puts on their relationships with family and loved ones. Faced with a medical system that is ill-equipped to properly diagnose and treat chronic and complex disorders, Tracey shows courage and tenacious determination to heal by taking the management of this "mystery illness" into her own hands. It is an inspiring must read for anyone dealing with chronic illness."

— CHRISTOPHER BUTLER, *Acupuncture and Functional Medicine*

"*Not My Buddy* leads the reader through Tracey's maze of health issues not cured by mainstream medicine. Using the Functional Medicine approach to her health issues Tracey was able to navigate her quest back to health. Functional Medicine is a personalized, systems-oriented model that empowers patients and practitioners to achieve the highest expression of health by working in collaboration to address the underlying causes of disease. Using the model in conjunction with tapping countless resources and 'erko's' emotional fortitude ushered the way to, spoiler alert, a healthy outcome."

— DANIEL ZACHARIAS, MD

"Having read an advanced copy of *Not My Buddy*, I was blown away by Tracey's deeply personal and wise story."

— ROLIN SAN JUAN, *Owner, Bodies inMotion Wellness Studio*

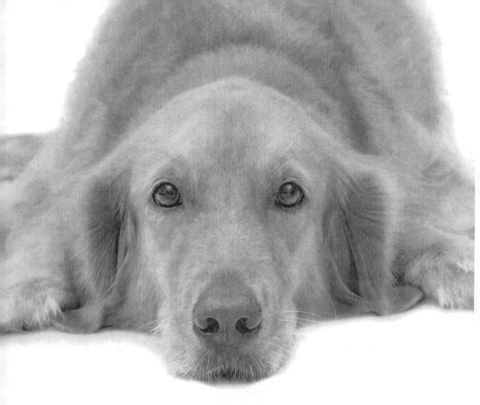

NOT MY BUDDY

One woman, a dog,
and their journey
toward healing

TRACEY BERKOWITZ

GEMINI

Published in the United States by Gemini Press, New Jersey

GEMINI

FIRST EDITION

Berkowitz, Tracey.
Not My Buddy: One woman, a dog,
and their journey toward healing

ISBN #978-0-9907355-0-2 (pbk)
ISBN #978-0-9907355-1-9 (hc)
ISBN #978-0-9907355-2-6 (eb)

Library of Congress Control Number: 2014917747

Printed in the United States of America

Cover and Interior design by Tom Joyce/Creativewerks
Author's photo by Nicole Dersovitz

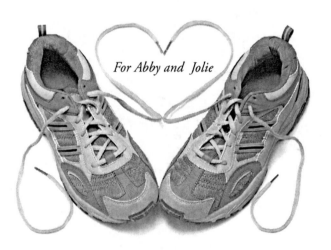

For Abby and Jolie

*"2.5 million cases of giardiasis
occur each year in the United States,
and up to 20% of the world's population
are chronically infected."*

– STATED ON cdc.gov.

FOREWORD

LEO GALLAND, M.D.
THE FOUNDATION FOR INTEGRATED MEDICINE
NEW YORK, NEW YORK

CHRONIC GIARDIASIS is a devastating illness that starts with digestive symptoms but can spread to impact your whole body. Fatigue, allergies, skin rashes, swollen lymph glands, muscle pain and arthritis can follow. Giardia infection may cause an overgrowth of yeast or bacteria in the small intestine, producing another infectious source of symptoms that doesn't go away just because the giardia parasite is treated. It's a nightmare for patients and a challenge for doctors.

Tracey Berkowitz guides us through her nightmare with humor and grace. The first challenge is making a diagnosis. The lab tests are imperfect and despite the high prevalence of giardia infection in the U.S., the notion that giardia is primarily a travel-related illness is pervasive. The second challenge is treatment. Although effective drugs are available, they often don't cure the illness, for either of two reasons: reinfection and persistence.

Giardia infection is readily transmitted within families. Living together, preparing food, sharing bathrooms and bedrooms, and intimate contact. The cyst of giardia is a robust survivor and remains infectious on surfaces like doorknobs for two weeks.

Both the cure of giardia and the development of symptoms are not primarily determined by the parasite, but by the immune system of its human host. If you suffer from giardiasis, most of the damage, whether it occurs in the small intestines where giardia lives, or in the skin and joints, where there are no parasites, results from the actions of your own immune system. This is a paradox that can be hard to wrap your mind around, because it takes the activity of the same immune system to eliminate giardia all together. The antibiotics just weaken the bug. You have to kill it off. When you add to this seeming contraction the fact some people may harbor the same parasite with no ill effects—they're just carriers—the full mystery of giardiasis emerges. There is nothing simple about this illness.

Tracey shares her frustrations and her persistence with you. Her drive to restore her life to normal helped her transform her life and gave her a new mission, helping others with chronic giardiasis find ways to restore their own health.

CHAPTER
1

I N APRIL 2009, I stood in front of a full-length mirror and stared at my distended belly. I'd given birth to twin girls eight years earlier but looked and felt as if I was about to go into labor, except I was not pregnant. What I was—was a mystery. My runner's body had vanished overnight. I struggled to stay balanced on my feet. My dark hair, once shiny, had turned dull and fell out in clumps. I was shedding as frequently as the Golden Retriever that sat at my feet. Something was very wrong and he knew it. Buddy stared up at me, yearning for attention and a chance to play, but any activity other than sleep was more than I could handle. He was barely a year old, but I swear he was trying to apologize. His big brown eyes asked, *is it really my fault?*

🐾 🐾

My fraternal twin daughters, Abby and Jolie, begged me to get a dog after we read every tale of *Biscuit the Puppy* and watched all the "Air Bud" movies. By May 2008, my husband and I finally gave in and contacted the breeder that my sister used the prior year. We told the girls we were going to the "dog farm," the breeder's house, to play with purebred Golden Retrievers.

I melted seeing the girls sitting on the kennel floor surrounded by a new litter. I didn't care that it was filthy—it was a kennel after all. Abby and Jolie were ecstatic.

"What would you say if we told you that we can bring one of these puppies home soon?"

A chorus of *"OMGs"* were followed by a round of *"THANK YOUs!"*

Two weeks later, we returned to choose our puppy.

Choosing a puppy required some preparation and a lot of reading. I had done my homework, determined to find just the right dog for our family. What exactly did that mean? I wanted a smart dog, an affectionate dog, a dog that behaved and was good with children and made bad people run like hell from our house. I wanted a dog that looked cute, that we loved very much and that loved us back unconditionally. I wanted a dog that the girls would learn to take care of. Like a 4-H project. We could do this, I kept telling myself. It might even be fun.

I did not have a dog growing up and hadn't considered myself a dog person until I spent time at my first boyfriend's house in junior high school. Stephen owned a beautiful blonde Golden Retriever with a seemingly submissive personality. He made it look like taking care of a dog was easy. I thought so, too, until his dog pinned me against the door in Stephen's laundry room, where he stayed when people visited. All he wanted was to play with someone and receive some attention. I knew he wouldn't hurt me but I panicked and screamed for help.

Later in college, I had another chance to become a dog lover when my roommate agreed to keep her boyfriend's new litter of Bulldog puppies at our apartment. Their hairless bodies fit into the palms of our hands and I found myself racing home from class every day to play with them. Once they were sold, our apartment seemed empty. I was startled by how quickly I had bonded with those puppies and I missed them very much.

When my daughters fell in love with the storybook character "Biscuit," it didn't take much time for me to start dreaming about our new lives together. I could imagine myself in our local dog park, chatting with my new dog lover friends, tossing Frisbees and balls, comparing dog foods and obedience training. Adding a dog to our family would complete us, I believed. The picture was almost perfect. I wanted 'the perfect dog,' but every puppy squirmed right out of my arms before I could complete the four personality tests recommended in *Good Owners, Great Dogs; What All Good Dogs Should Know; Children with their Dogs* and *Golden Retrievers for Dummies.*

"You think those tests will work completely?" my husband, Jeff, asked dubiously. I continued petting the puppy between my legs, aware of my husband's smirking.

I refused to let his healthy skepticism alter my plans. He nudged me a few times in the arm, then flashed his goofy, dimpled grin and raised his eyebrows until they disappeared under the lid of his baseball hat. He raised his hat in one hand, pushed back his brown hair with the other and winked—as if to emphasize his teasing. I elbowed him and rolled my eyes.

The breeder helped narrow the selection for us, removing the puppies we didn't want, leaving us with three males whose fur wouldn't get thick like a wolf. We didn't want to ruin the carpets for God's sake.

Abby insisted we take the runt. "He is so calm and not biting my shoelaces like the other ones. He's small and cute like me," she said and smiled.

"No way I'm taking the runt!" I declared. I wanted a healthy dog. Maybe even a show dog. A dog we could rally behind, the centerpiece of holiday cards. Abby flipped me a look.

"How about this one," Jolie asked. "He's cute and sort of calm." She laughed when he jumped right out of her arms and looked at us. "I guess. It's so hard to choose."

Jeff held one of the puppies for a while. The puppy seemed calm. Jeff turned the puppy on his back to cradle him—using the personality test he had mocked. "Trace, he's really sweet and he's been hanging out in my arms the longest. We're never going to know what any of these pups will be like in a few months. We'll train him and he'll be great. Take him."

I grabbed onto the six-pound bundle of fur. He was sweet and looked directly into my eyes. I turned him over, rubbing my hand around his little bald belly, feeling the warmth and softness. It struck me, here's my chance to have a third child—despite his performance on those personality tests. Suddenly, I forgot about the books. My future pulsed with possibility. It was as if I'd finally get to experience what caring for a newborn "baby" would be like without the constant worry of splitting my attention equally like I had always done with the twins.

I paused with my hand over his heart and scratched under his chin. He hardly moved, clearly relishing this connection. Cradled on his back, he didn't squirm much, and he nipped only playfully. Clearly, this was a gentle soul wrapped in just the right amount of soft blond fur. He passed all four tests. I glanced at my family. "I can't believe I am going to say this, but I like him. I think he's the one! I think we found our Buddy guys!"

At ten weeks old, Buddy would be ready to leave his mother and siblings and start a new life with us. We gave the breeder a deposit and returned Memorial Day Weekend to pick up Buddy. While I filled out the last of the paperwork, the breeder told us that Buddy had a parasite.

I paused and looked up at him. "A parasite?"

The breeder shrugged and nodded. "Yeah, giardia. It's very common among puppies. Nothing that this won't cure," he said and handed me a Ziploc bag with tubes of liquid antibiotics, instructing us to inject them into his mouth every day for a week. His relaxed manner eliminated the need to inquire further. I figured parasites, especially in puppies, were no big deal, like my girls having the stomach flu.

"Easy, right?" he asked.

I nodded, recalling the times I gave Jolie acid reflux medicine when she was an infant, and within a few days her stomach got better. I could handle this.

We took more pictures and headed home while my daughters bickered over who got to have Buddy on her lap. I refused to let anything ruin our beautiful day and sat in the back seat between them while Buddy laid on my lap, completing the perfect picture.

Later that afternoon, Jeff and I stood on our deck, watching Buddy interact with our girls in the backyard. Jolie sat on the grass Indian-style, with her dirty blonde hair in a low ponytail, her back against the tree, coddling Buddy. She looked more relaxed and confident than I had ever seen her. Caring for an animal came naturally to her, and she clearly appreciated Buddy's attention after years of sharing everything with her fraternal twin. I was amazed that Jolie kept up with him after hours of play. Her intentions from the start were genuine. She was looking for a companion in this puppy.

Abby had a slightly different experience. She enjoyed Buddy's attention when she was in the mood to play with him, establishing a more conditional love. When Abby decided to move on to something else, such as the swing set, she expected Buddy to leave her alone, but he nipped at her clothing. Abby was frustrated, so I sat her down on the grass and tried to help.

I gently swept away Abby's thick brown hair behind each ear, revealing her tiny face and light brown eyes. "You have to ignore him when he nips at you. It's a puppy's way of teething and playing. If you keep moving every time he does it, he will do it again. It's a game for him."

Abby's eyes welled up with tears. "It's annoying. Why doesn't he do that with you guys or Jolie? We should have picked the runt," she said, crossing her arms. "Besides, you like him more than me."

"Oh Ab," I said with a slight chuckle. She couldn't possibly believe I would favor a dog over her. I continued, "Come on. You don't really believe that? You're my sweetheart, and I love you so much, but we just brought a puppy home who needs to be watched at all times. This is the part about being responsible that Daddy and I discussed with you girls. Remember? We have to train him and teach him how to be a well-behaved dog."

"Buddy likes you guys better than me," Abby said between gasps. Tears ran down her face. I wrapped my arms around her.

"Buddy is just looking for attention and will take it from anyone who gives it. Why don't you go inside the house and grab a treat," I offered. "Next time he deserves a reward, I'll let you be the one to give it. Trust me, he'll remember who gave him the good stuff and come back for more!"

House-training Buddy demanded even more of our attention. By the third day, the only thing I was scrubbing was his poop off the terra cotta tile floor in my kitchen. While I was on my knees, I wondered if I was really cut out for this. I had never felt more ex-

hausted, and yet only three weeks ago, I had run a half marathon.
I wondered if we should have gotten the runt.

Jolie pointed out the spreading mess, "Uh mom, he made over
here, too."

"You've got to be kidding me!" I said, convinced I had picked
the wrong puppy.

After Memorial Day Weekend, I was left alone with Buddy. Jeff
was back at work and the girls were off to school. Buddy explored
the kitchen while I sat at the table, dressed in gym clothes, yearning to go on my morning run. Since Buddy cried the first couple
of nights in his crate, we didn't sleep very well, although no one
else in my family seemed to be affected. Their energy was intact.
I attributed my fatigue to the stress of being responsible for this
new puppy. However, my exhaustion from caring for infant twins
didn't compare to what I felt like now, and I had spent only a
couple days with him. This should have been a cakewalk, but I
could barely lift my head off the table.

I noticed Buddy slow down as he approached the corner
below the kitchen island. It was obvious he was about to make
another mess. I shut my eyes for a brief moment and sighed.

"Just fabulous, Buddy."

I should have swept him up, run outside, and used his bathroom command, "go hurry ups," but I did nothing. I was on
my knees cleaning his mess once again. I felt a lump in my throat
and an uneasy sensation in my stomach, this time attributing it to
constipation, knowing it had almost been two days since I'd gone
to the bathroom. I fought tears as I cleaned Buddy's mess. I didn't
recall my sister complaining too much about raising Jagger, her
Golden Retriever, which she had affectionately called her "third
child." How could I feel so tortured by our adorable puppy?

The telephone rang. At first, I didn't get up to answer it. I had no desire to speak to anyone and give them the opportunity to ask how things were, because I was embarrassed that I couldn't handle this simple situation. My machine picked up and I waited to hear the message.

"Hi Tracey. This is Debbie returning your call. When you get a minute."

Thank God, I thought. It was the dog trainer to rescue me.

I struggled to get off the floor and dove for the telephone before she hung up.

"Thank you for returning my call. I am so happy to hear your voice!" I said, a little breathless. "You have no idea. I need serious help. My dog is having accidents all over the place and I'm exhausted and miserable. When can you come?"

Debbie listened to my desperate pleas for help and calmly redirected my focus. She explained that Buddy was acting as *my* master, when the roles should be reversed. She wrapped up our half hour call, explaining that we would start lessons when he was twelve weeks old.

I could barely wait. Until our first appointment, I listened to her instructions as if my life depended on it. She told me to get him on a leash and follow him in circles outside until he went to the bathroom after I said my command, *hurry ups.* If he didn't go after a few minutes, I should bring him back into the house and put him immediately in the crate. When I was ready to take him out of the crate and try again, I should repeat the whole routine in the same spot with his leash: command, praise and treat. CPT, I told myself. It wasn't that hard. Then I was supposed to let him back into the kitchen, but at no time should I let him roam around the house.

"Keep him in a confined area," Debbie reminded me. "You are the master, not him. Make that clear and you'll be fine. He is following your lead. I'll see you in two weeks as originally agreed."

I scribbled down her tips as fast as I could so I wouldn't forget anything. I was grateful for Debbie's instructions. Crate training meant I could put the puppy in the crate even while I was home. Somehow I missed that important detail even after reading all four books.

A week later, I had become Buddy's master. I had even gotten used to our new schedule, but was still feeling constipated and extremely fatigued. Jeff and my mom agreed. "You're probably getting run-down from Buddy and should take something so you can go to the bathroom." I wish it could have been as simple as using a laxative or any such remedy. It had been a week since I had relief and the size of my belly was the proof. I looked like I was starting a second trimester of pregnancy, and what I was about to give birth to remained a huge mystery.

Saturday afternoon, I joined Jeff in the backyard while he laid on a lounge chair. Buddy ran in circles while the girls played on the swing set. I waved, forcing a smile. It was great to see everyone in such good spirits, but I was feeling crummy. They waved me over to join them.

"Sorry, girls. I just need a little break," I said, catching Jeff's eye. I rarely turned down the chance to join the girls for any kind of play, especially when I was training for the marathon. I welcomed any physical activity to stay pumped with endorphins; however, the most exercise I'd gotten lately consisted of bending down to clean up after Buddy.

Jeff flashed me a look of disbelief as I feigned relaxing on the lounge chair, face turned up to the sun with a pained smile. My bulging stomach felt like someone had put a vice around it. I shifted on the lounge chair, trying to find a better position until I could no longer ignore the discomfort. I finally confessed to Jeff. "I really don't feel right. It's been like this all week, especially now.

Something's wrong. I think I need to go to the emergency room."

Jeff wasn't too surprised by my news but dreaded the ER visit. He was running a small company and had to pay for our health insurance himself. Any extra out of pocket medical appointments would deplete our monthly budget. Hospitals scared him to death for good reason. It had taken us a while to recover from our infertility expenses and the complications that went along with the twins' birth. At the start of my pregnancy, we found ourselves in the ER every week. I either needed IVs, relieving extreme dehydration that my around the clock 'morning sickness' caused, or took tests that confirmed I wasn't going into pre-term labor. Each time I laid on the gurney in those ER cubicles, I stared at the walls, fixating on the high-risk pregnancy that was distressing my body and worried for the health of my babies. If it wasn't my sister waiting with me, it was Jeff, who found solace in the chair nearby, aimlessly channel surfing the television stations. During most visits, the majority of long hours were spent in silence, coping with our fears. Clearly, the hospital was the last place that Jeff wanted to visit with me.

"If you think you need to go, then let's go. You know your body best. I mean your stomach does look sort of... huge," he said staring, incredulous, at my belly. I knew what I looked like but his acknowledgement stung. I worked hard at maintaining my body size.

We canceled our dinner plans and spent the night in the emergency room instead.

CHAPTER
2

M UCH TO JEFF'S DISMAY, I had to complete all the required tests and body scans. The doctor attributed my constipation to not eating regular meals or drinking enough water during the week. "I ordered an enema," he said. "The nurse should be here any minute. You'll feel much better once you're relieved. We will watch you to make sure it does the trick before you go home."

After all this time, an enema was all I needed? His explanation did not add up.

"How could I look like this from a change of food and lack of water intake in just one week?" I offered my own theories. "We just got a puppy last weekend. Is it possible I am allergic to him?" I asked, suddenly recalling the conversation with my sister after we brought Buddy home. When I mentioned the breeder supplied us with medication for parasites, she wasn't concerned because her dog also had this parasite and she left the breeder's property with the same antibiotics. Was this a mere coincidence? Even though no one in her family got sick, I felt like this was important information to share. "Oh, wait, he also has some sort of parasite named, uh, giardia. Could I have gotten that?"

The doctor's beeper went off. He grabbed it from his belt buckle, glanced at the message and looked back at me. "Your dog should have nothing to do with this situation. Humans don't typically get that from dogs and your symptoms don't match up either. We'll get you better before you leave. I am sure you are frustrated and tired at this point. I'll be back once you take the enema and let's see where you're at."

Jeff saw my face fall and knew I wasn't satisfied. After the first enema was unsuccessful, the doctor ordered a second one. While waiting for this one to work, I wracked my brain for a better explanation. I came up with nothing, banking on the doctor's expertise.

Neither enema procedures relieved my symptoms and only caused more discomfort in my abdomen. I was too sick to ask why I had not improved. The doctor ordered a third enema and a hospital room.

"Once you get transferred, the nurse upstairs will give it to you. You should see your internist during rounds tomorrow morning in case you have further questions. Good luck and feel better."

I was not feeling better, but it was a comfort to have Jeff by my side for a while. I encouraged him to go home and relieve the babysitter. "There's no point to sit here with me while I wait to be transferred. I'll be sure to text you if I explode. Besides, I don't want the girls to worry about me. And, someone has to deal with Buddy."

Jeff planted a kiss on my lips before leaving the emergency room cubicle.

"I love you, hon. If you can, try to get a decent sleep and I'll call you in the morning. Hang in there...and oh, good luck with that explosion!" he said and winked.

Once I was transferred to the second floor of the hospital, the nurse reminded me, "Third time's the charm sweetie." I had high hopes for relief. Within minutes, I felt the kind of pressure inside me as if someone turned on the faucet to a backyard hose. I grabbed the bathroom side rail to keep my balance and prayed for good aim. I was sweating profusely and losing my balance. My body was growing weaker by the second and my hands trembled, and I wondered why we ever got Buddy.

I bristled hearing my internist's response the next morning.

"I hear you finally had some relief last night. That must have felt good. Now what do you think happened for you to have experienced such severe constipation?"

I briefly reviewed my week, emphasizing my new puppy, the parasite he had and the many symptoms that led to my situation. The doctor was silent, then recommended I exercise more and stop taking Advil, which I had taken to relieve the onset of headaches. He closed my chart, stood and said, "I'll put you on a laxative for a short time so you can get back on schedule. Let's chalk it up to one action that spiraled into the next. You'll be fine."

CHAPTER
3

A FEW LICKS AND HUGS from Buddy was all I needed to lift my spirits. I threw myself into training him the rest of the summer in between a part-time job where I worked as an assistant teacher for two-year olds at a nearby pre-school. No matter what I had planned for the day, I always raced home for Buddy. Despite the minor fatigue and constipation, I didn't let it stop me from working with his trainer every ten days while my girls went to day camp. We focused on basic commands and practiced every day, hoping Buddy could impress Debbie.

Debbie was known as a "drill sergeant" because of her "rough around the edges" first impression; however, she had a compassionate side that I assumed anyone would see if they stuck to her regimen. I was inspired by her ability to communicate effortlessly with Buddy.

The minute Debbie arrived, Buddy knew she meant business. I shared my training accomplishments and Buddy's pitfalls. He jumped on guests, and I was worried that he would dart out the front door, too, because the front lawn wasn't fenced. Debbie recognized my commitment towards training Buddy and took her coaching to a new level.

Each morning after the girls left for camp, Buddy and I managed to walk a few miles throughout the neighborhood despite my fatigue. I always made sure to lead so I used a prong collar. When he got ahead of me, I yanked the collar to remind him I was his master.

"Make sure to get enough treats in your hand," Debbie reminded me one day, taking Buddy fifteen feet away from me so he would not get distracted.

I envied the respect he had for her, and stood, mouth agape, watching Buddy run fifty feet toward her after hearing her stern voice. "BUDDY COME…HERE." She pointed her finger towards the grass in front of her. Like clockwork, Buddy stopped inches from her feet and sat motionless with his eyes solely focused on hers. The drill sergeant had done it. I was in awe of her leadership. It didn't matter if I had a fist full of treats, Buddy would never stop like that for me.

After several hours of practice, we managed to get a decent amount of distance between us; however, I was still concerned that he didn't listen when distracted, especially when he saw other dogs. I was also worried that he wasn't social enough, after a friend mentioned this phenomena. "Social?" I asked, staring at her wide-eyed. She nodded emphatically. I seriously considered signing Buddy up for a puppy socialization class, but because he still had giardia, we met Debbie instead for our next lesson at the beautiful Verona Park, close to town.

🐾 🐾

Debbie chose the most crowded spots at the park as a way to test Buddy, but she always kept some distance between him and the other dogs. We worked hard to keep Buddy's attention focused only on the sound of my voice, though he clearly responded more to hers.

After enough practice, I was eager to move on to the next command, "stay." Buddy's ears perked up every time he heard a noise while his eyes moved side-to-side. I wanted to laugh, witnessing his responses, and thought I should pay attention and live in the moment like him. Like a baby, he was tuned into the birds and the bees and the trees and the grass, anything and everything but me. He was also enjoying this training much more than me. Clearly, I was the student here and my lessons in true presence had only just begun.

Once Buddy stayed on the ground long enough and ignored distractions like an infant's cry or a stranger's conversation, I rewarded him with a small treat. "Who's a good boy?" I asked, petting his face. I glanced back at Debbie and asked, "Can you get him to stay like this at my front door next session? It would be nice to open the door more than just a crack without his nose forced between my legs." I wondered if she would help me control his bowels, too.

Buddy's parasite lasted through the summer. One afternoon, after I dropped off his latest stool sample at the vet to get retested for giardia, we went to Petco for more puppy food. I figured he'd be fine to come inside the store because he'd gone to the bathroom before we left the house.

I recalled the days of potty training the girls, when I kept a spare potty in the trunk for close calls, which were easier to handle with toddlers than a sick puppy whose only way of communicating was scratching at the kitchen door.

As I swiped my credit card at Petco, Buddy's leash tugged at my wrist. I looked over to see him squatting on the floor producing Willy Wonka's chocolate stream. My first reaction was to bolt as soon as I got my receipt. I looked up at the clerk, horrified.

"Uh, my dog just had an accident on your floor. I didn't know if there is someone that I should tell in order to clean up the mess?"

"You see the wipes and bags right at the end of the counter? That's what you can use to clean it up," the cashier said without the faintest smile.

I looked down at Buddy next to his pile, his eyebrows raised as he looked at me.

I grabbed some wipes and knelt down cursing under my breath, stuffing as much as I could into the bag. I whispered, "Seriously Bud? Come on!" I didn't say a word to him the whole way home and wondered what kind of hell I had entered by getting a puppy.

Later that night, Jeff gave Buddy his medication, sensing my agitation and waning patience. On those nights, I became short tempered and needed space to recover from incidents that would have hardly bothered me when the girls were infants. By comparison, I would have chosen sleep deprivation over cleaning Buddy's messes at home or in public, or worse, getting him to acknowledge that I was his *master*. I suddenly wished he was a baby, not a puppy—at least he couldn't bolt out the door. I had this sinking feeling that Buddy didn't need me as much as I needed him—for what, I still did not know. Though I had a dog now, dog ownership certainly wasn't the perfect picture I envisioned it to be. I was definitely not a dog lover yet.

Buddy was testing me on every level, especially when it came time to take his medication. He was on his third round of Flagyl, an antibiotic to treat the giardia, but refused to take the pill without a scene. After Petco, I couldn't handle any more of his disobedience.

"Use the peanut butter," I said. "This morning, he spit the pill out even after he finished the piece of cheese that I hid it in. With his pills, he's a genius. At Petco—not so much!"

"Boo, you're not going to do that to me, right?" Jeff stood by the kitchen sink and prepared the spoonful of peanut butter. He hid the pill so Buddy couldn't see it. "Ok, who's a good boy?" Buddy started to lick the spoon. He continued, "You like that right?" When Buddy got to the area where the pill was hidden, he stopped, tilted his head and stared back at Jeff. Jeff fixed what was left of the peanut butter and covered the pill yet again. Buddy licked a few more times, stopped and sat down. He waited for Jeff's next move. "Would you look at this dog?"

I locked eyes with Buddy, catching what I believed to be a bona fide puppy smirk. Our puppy was only three months old but acting like a teenager. How could this happen? Wasn't he sensing my love and devotion? Maybe not. Deep down, I could not wait to take a break from puppy duty when I would take the girls to Cancun and stay with my parents at one of their timeshare condominiums. Jeff had to stay at home because of work and agreed to take care of Buddy. I had no objections. Mexico, I believed, would make me feel better.

CHAPTER
4

I HOPED FOR MONTEZUMA'S REVENGE in Mexico to relieve my constipation. Though I was free from Buddy, I struggled to keep my exercise regimen. My four-mile runs became two, and by the end of the week, I barely finished a mile. I'm not even sure I would have been able to take Buddy for a walk. My parents were disturbed by these changes and my dependence on laxatives.

I was just as baffled, knowing my body endured five months of training that accompanied my first half-marathon that year. I was used to exercising religiously seven days a week, starting at sunrise on our basement elliptical for forty-five minutes and continuing on the gym treadmill for another two hours after I dropped the girls off at school. Twice a week, I finished the cardio portion of my workouts with a trainer, lifting weights, jumping rope, using various skipping styles and even excelled at traveling plank claps. My workouts weren't complete unless I left the gym covered in sweat. Clearly, lack of willpower was not the culprit. Raising twins from birth had taught me endurance; however, by the last meal of our trip to Mexico, my parents urged me to confront my situation.

"Your diet is pristine and I don't know anyone who eats more roughage than you," my mother said, reminding me that I ate a salad twice a day and egg whites every morning. How much more could I eat or take out of my diet without starving myself?

"I think it's time to see your gynecologist," she said, reminding me I still hadn't gotten my period after the half marathon. My father was equally concerned, "Maybe the bloat is related to those other symptoms. Do us a favor please, make an appointment."

I nodded, hoping to move on to more pleasant conversations. "A friend recommended a nutritionist who helped her with similar symptoms. I'll see her as soon as I get home."

A week after vacation, I met Kathy, the nutritionist, in her office on a Sunday morning. I reviewed my recent turn of events, emphasizing the bloat and minor weight gain around my abdomen and now my parents' concerns, which were not yet my own. The truth is that life without menstruating was a lot easier on me, considering the new role I'd taken on training Buddy and cleaning up his own mess. Kathy encouraged me to have my gynecologist do a full panel of blood work to make sure I wasn't deficient in any areas.

"There are other options if you have to fix your hormones, but you can't pretend a problem doesn't exist," she said. Then she gave her qualifications of being a Life Coach and explained how her six-month program worked. We would meet every ten days during which time she would introduce another food group that naturally heals and balances the body. Kathy emphasized the importance of releasing your emotions to live a stress-free life no matter what.

That sounded good to me. It didn't take a doctor or any professional to make me aware that I was already stressed out. "I'm definitely interested and would love to work with you," I said. "A stress-free life while raising kids, and a puppy…that would be wonderful, if true."

Kathy gave me a thoughtful glance.

"Have you ever tried meditation before? It really helps clear your mind and is another way people heal their bodies."

I chuckled. "I took a few hot yoga classes, does that count?" I asked, wondering if downward dog would be enough to center me. "I figured all that sweat helped with weight loss."

Kathy held my gaze, without judgment, then handed me the appropriate paperwork to sign and an empty notebook to fill during our six months together.

Then she got up and grabbed a CD from her bookshelf. "Try this meditation CD before your next appointment. All you need is a half hour of quiet time but if you don't like this one, I have others to try next time we meet." I took the CD and dropped it in my bag, wondering when I'd find those sacred thirty minutes. All this sounded great in theory, but so far, theory had not translated well to early parenthood—or puppyhood. Each day presented new lessons, a sort of Whack-A-Mole that I had learned to play. I felt the stress meter spike as I walked out the door.

One week later, the opportunity presented itself to give this 'quiet time' a chance. The girls had a two-hour birthday party, and Jeff agreed to take them, leaving Buddy and me with roughly three hours to ourselves.

I turned the den lights off and grabbed the *Chakra Visualization* CD from the coffee table. Buddy's eyes followed my every move.

I pressed play and heard a xylophone and a harp. I went back to the couch, laid down and waited for "the silence" to work. Buddy's ears perked up and he gave me a wink. "Ready for a stress-free life?" He stared back at me. "I know it's weird but I said I would give it a shot, so try to enjoy it and don't bother me until it's over."

Just then a woman began to speak. Her tone was soft and precise. "Make sure you are lying down somewhere that's comfortable. Close your eyes and begin to take deep breaths in through your nose, hold it for four seconds and release all the negative thoughts out through your mouth." She explained the seven chakras, what they represent, how they relate to one another and the importance of keeping this spiral-like energy flowing freely throughout each center. This type of meditation helps to balance and activate the body's healing process. The minute my mind drifted, I reminded myself to follow her directions and focus on my breath.

I woke up abruptly when the telephone rang. It was dark in the den since it was nearly dinnertime. My body was so relaxed that it took me a few seconds to answer the phone. Jeff said, "We are on our way back, about fifteen minutes from home. The girls ate dinner at the party. You want me to pick up something for you?"

I mumbled, "Dinner, wow I guess I slept a while. I used that meditation CD when you left. God, I wonder where Buddy is?" I turned my head and saw the glare of his eyes. "OMG Jeff, he didn't move this entire time either, I am cracking up. Maybe we should wire this CD to play meditation sounds when someone rings the doorbell."

Jeff laughed, "That crazy dog." Buddy propped his head on his front paws and raised his eyebrows with a quizzical look. I couldn't wait to tell Kathy. So far, I liked her theory.

CHAPTER
5

I SAW MY GYNECOLOGIST three weeks after Kathy encouraged me to do my blood work. He focused solely on the disappearance of my period and didn't ask any more questions regarding the rest of my health. We discussed different options, but the doctor's first choice was to take Provera in order to bring on my period, suggesting birth control as a second option.

"The estrogen levels in the pills are very different these days. It shouldn't affect you as in the past."

He was very aware of my college experience at Ohio State University Hospital where I was told I had either an ulcer or cyst on my ovaries that needed to be surgically removed. My mother intervened and brought me home to see her doctor. He determined I was allergic to birth control pills, and within a month of stopping them, I felt better.

I was hesitant to try birth control again, but agreed with my gynecologist's recommendation. I fully trusted him after he safely delivered my twins just shy of my thirty-fifth week of pregnancy. After two-years of infertility medicines and procedures, I used a Reglan pump, which helps prevent vomiting in cancer patients, while I battled sixteen weeks of morning sickness. I also took Breathine pills to control pre-term labor contractions at twenty-one weeks. I had confidence in his recommendations.

I got the test results at dinner time a few days later. The OBGYN prescribed Provera based on my results. He mentioned that if I didn't get my period within fourteen days he would prescribe the lowest estrogen birth control pill. When I hung up, I returned to the kitchen table and shared this information with Jeff. "I am getting a second opinion."

Two weeks later, I did not get my period but consulted with two reputable reproductive gynecologists. Both doctors commented on my exercise routine and weight gain. "You probably lost your period due to the heavy exercise regimen" and agreed the weight gain was necessary. At five foot one and a half inches, I was a size two and weighed one hundred and nine pounds, staying within the correct guidelines according to Weight Watchers. Though I'd been on diets for much of my adult life, I cherished my body most at this weight and fixated on it.

CHAPTER
6

B Y OCTOBER, I started the LoEstrin birth control pill with few side effects until Thanksgiving. A few days before the holiday, I woke after a nap and heard laughter in the den, discovering the girls and Jeff playing with Buddy. At six months old, he was full of energy. I wanted to join their fun but felt as if a Mack truck had hit me. No matter how sleep deprived I was when the girls were first born, I never experienced exhaustion to this degree. I propped myself against the wall and continued to watch my family. Jolie held one of Buddy's chew toys as he tugged and pulled with his teeth, while Jeff was on all fours, his baseball hat rested on the carpet. Buddy growled with delight, loving the attention. Abby rode on Jeff's back, her thick brown hair covering most of her petite face as usual.

Jolie noticed my shadow in the background and shouted, "Buddy, mommy's up!" His head did not turn and he continued to play with his sister. Buddy had gotten used to my many disappearing acts. While I spent most of the time asleep, he bonded with Jeff, who had now become his master, much to my dismay. I had wanted that role, reasoning I should be the 'fun guy' since I was home most of the time, but it was gone.

"Hi, mommy. Did you have a good nap?" Jeff asked.

I walked directly to the couch and plopped myself down.

"Mommy, look at me. I'm getting a horsey ride from daddy!" Abby was all smiles, appreciating her father's attention. I barely grinned.

Jolie chimed in. "And I'm next. Right dad? Mom, you should have seen before, Buddy was humping Abby's leg again!"

"And yours too, Jolie," Abby responded firmly, reminding me of Buddy's appointment to be neutered the week we return from our upcoming trip.

Having no energy to react to anyone's comments, I looked toward Jeff. "I'm just so tired, nothing helps me feel better. I'm a walking zombie and I gained fifteen pounds."

Jeff stopped playing. "I know nothing about this Life Coach and the holistic foods you're eating, but is it possible that's what's making it worse?" Jeff waited for my response. When I rolled my eyes and shrugged my shoulders, he changed tactics, suggesting that our vacation in Belize would be the perfect opportunity to rest. Jeff and his college friend, Dave, found a modest resort that offered a relatively inexpensive deal for a five-night stay over Thanksgiving weekend, using our credit card points for two free flights.

Buddy brushed his paw against Jeff's arm enough times to get his attention since he wanted more playtime. Jeff looked back at Buddy, "What, you want some more of this?"

While Jeff played with Buddy, I wondered how everything would get accomplished before our upcoming trip—and I hated having to lean on others for help. I watched my family enjoy our puppy, as I lay motionless on the den couch.

CHAPTER
7

N O MATTER HOW MUCH we laughed and enjoyed time with our friends in Belize, my health was always the elephant in the room. After Jeff and I returned from vacation, dinner conversations revolved around my health and were constantly interrupted by phone calls from doctors. I had been taking the birth control pill for almost three months, getting my period on a regular basis and yet, my health plummeted. I looked like I was in my third trimester and I was very scared.

Abby shouted as I picked up the phone to speak with my gynecologist, "Not again, Dad! She's always on the phone now."

I shared my new symptoms with the doctor and walked toward the den, hearing Jeff respond to Abby's comment.

"Mommy really doesn't feel well now. We have to be patient with her. I know it's hard but she needs to speak to the doctors so she can find out what's wrong and how to get better."

"But we never get time with her anymore," Jolie said. "It's always about her sickness."

I stood in the den, listening to the doctor. He wasn't convinced my elevated hormones and bloating were related and didn't support the use of natural remedies or stopping the pill to see if my symptoms would change. "I think it's time you see a gastroenterologist," he said.

It took a moment for his response to sink in before I returned to the kitchen table and sat in the chair next to Jeff, using my arm to prop up my head and hide the fatigue from the girls. I motioned for the girls to clean up their place setting from the table once they finished eating. Abby got up to throw what was left of her dinner in the garbage while I shared the doctor's opinions. She turned to me as tears fell down her cheeks. "Are you going to die?" she asked. I gasped.

My eyes filled with tears while she walked over. I grabbed her hands and pulled her close between my legs, "Oh my god, Abby. Of course not. This must seem scary to you and I am sorry both you girls have to watch me like this." I looked over at Jolie, who stood motionless and continued, "I don't know what's wrong yet and that's why I am talking to so many doctors. I'm sorry if you think I am not around, but I promise you I will do everything I can to get better. I am not going anywhere! I promise!" I said, acknowledging that I heard her earlier discussion with Jeff. I then wiped her tears and hugged her tightly, praying I could keep this promise.

Later that night, Jeff shared some of his concerns in the privacy of our bedroom. "It's crazy she thought you would die. You never know what's going through those little minds." After hearing Abby's comment, I decided to be more discreet when Jeff and I discussed the doctors and the status of my health. I lowered my voice and made sure the door was closed completely.

"What if she's right?" I got choked up, but continued, "Nobody's helping me at this point. The doctor told me to just deal with it and I'm only getting worse. Look at me! I haven't exercised in months and I constantly miss work because I'm so tired. It's pathetic!"

Jeff got into bed and lay next to me.

I continued, "And I'm losing my hair."

Jeff turned to me and laughed. "You're what?"

"Don't laugh. I'm serious. Just the other day when I was showering, a huge clump fell out." After childbirth, I experienced hair loss around my temples like any woman does. I didn't really think about that much at the outset. But this shouldn't be happening.

"I think you're just stressed. Come here." He stretched his arm around my shoulders and pulled me into his chest. I knew he was trying to comfort me, but lately I felt undesirable from my body's changes and I cringed at his touch. And now I had issues with my hair, which was the only thing I always cherished about myself. Though he continued trying to hug me, I kept my arms at my sides and avoided eye contact, staring at the chipped paint on our bedroom wall.

"If he said to see a gastro doc, then that's what you'll do. Trust me, I see what you look like—obviously it's something. Someone's going to figure this out. I can't say much about your hair since mine's been falling out for years, but try not to worry." We both shared an awkward laugh. "Besides, look on the bright side, at least we are past Buddy losing his manhood and he doesn't have to wear that ridiculous looking lamp shade that we duct taped together after he banged into every kitchen cabinet." Jeff met my eyes, waiting for any expression. "Plus now *your* genius dog finally stopped humping everyone!"

I forced a smile and rolled over, blowing him a kiss goodnight, laying in the dark while twisting my thinning hair between my fingertips, wondering if I had cancer.

The next morning I dropped the girls off at school and drove to my therapist's office. I had been seeing her for a little over a year. It started as a way to ease my stress. Even when my life seemed great, I wasn't completely content, which left me searching for happiness elsewhere. Now my sickness monopolized every appointment; however, it comforted me to know this doctor was witnessing all my recent changes.

I updated her on my health condition and decided to meet her every week. Receiving her unbiased opinion on what to do next was important. Sue had the ability to get to the heart of each matter and focus on a new plan of attack. She knew I was not a fan of my current internist. Sue insisted my internist should take the lead on my case. "And if not him, then find a replacement," she advised. At the very least, she agreed with my gynecologist that it was time to see a gastroenterologist for the bloat.

Prior to this, the last time I had seen my internist was when my body couldn't fight an infection on its own, three weeks before the half marathon. I had walked into his office with a sinus infection and strep throat, and left with antibiotics and a warning: "You need to take at least a week off from your training in order for your body to heal."

What did I do? I went ahead and ran nine miles in the misty rain after drinking wine with friends the night before, then showed up in his office with pink eye. His warning turned into an ultimatum. "Do you want to end up in the hospital? It's either 72 hours of bed rest or miss the marathon altogether."

I saw my internist again two days later. While he examined me, I brought him up to speed. "My arms feel like lead, I'm spent and look as if I'm pregnant but I'm not—I'm taking the pill and it's still difficult to go to the bathroom, even with those laxatives you prescribed." I did not feel comfortable telling him that my libido had also diminished, assuming my fatigue caused the lack of intimacy in my bedroom.

He looked at my file again. Between his frustrated pen clicks, I offered another idea.

"Could it be hypothyroidism? I read online and have many of the same symptoms. I've gained fifteen pounds in such a short time."

He closed the file. "You have a busy lifestyle. I'm sure you're on the go a lot with your kids. Do you eat your meals standing up or find yourself stressed before you eat?"

My brows furrowed. "I'm busy with my girls but definitely sit down when eating most meals. Maybe I snack standing up, sometimes?" I said, then pointed to my distended belly. "But I never had this huge belly before and I've seen a holistic nutritionist for four months now, so it can't be my food."

He continued to click his pen.

"Maybe your brain is wired a certain way that it can't multi-task in this environment and you should move to Tahiti and live on Pina Coladas by the beach," he said without a smile.

I stared at him, incredulous, feeling my heart pound. "I've raised twins for over eight years, work part-time and take care of a dog. I would say that's multi-tasking! Could you at least draw blood to see if my thyroid is low?"

He nodded, "I'll draw blood and let you know if I find something. You might also have Irritable Bowel Syndrome. Try sitting down and relaxing before each snack or meal," he said, insisting on smaller bites of food, then handed me the form to have my blood taken.

🐾 🐾

My hands shook as I pushed the elevator button. I grabbed my cell phone from my bag and dialed Jeff at work. By the time I left the building and got to my car, I had recapped my appointment. Once I closed the door and sat in the drivers seat, I cried, wondering if the doctor was right. Was I causing my body to look and feel like this because I was stressed out?

Or was I just going insane?

Jeff waited until I was calm before he spoke. "Whether or not he was serious is beside the point. You didn't cause any of this and hopefully, we'll get some answers tomorrow at your gastro appointment." He wanted me to relax before I drove home. I didn't see how that was possible.

"I'm fine!" I said and jerked on the ignition, then put the car in reverse. "I'll talk to you later." I hung up then turned on my iPod, which lasted two traffic lights before I dialed my mother.

CHAPTER
8

WHILE I WAITED for the gastroenterologist to finish reviewing my chart, I noticed a number of spiritual quotes displayed throughout his office. One in particular caught my eye. *Find joy in the journey.* It was the same quote I received from Kathy when we discussed living a stress-free life. The nurse took blood while the doctor ordered a colonoscopy for the following Monday morning, which left me doing the prep work Sunday afternoon.

I was only twenty-four hours away from receiving answers. I took four Dulcolax tablets with a large bottle of Myralax and mixed them with sixty-four ounces of Crystal Light lemonade. I needed to finish the drink within two to three hours.

Jeff came to the bedroom periodically to check on me, surprised by what appeared to be an abnormal response to the prep work. He found me motionless and half awake with the large glass of liquid on my nightstand, half full. He approached my side of the bed.

"Are you supposed to be this weak?" he asked, seeing my pale face.

I could hardly tilt my head towards Jeff and whimpered. "It's coming out of me from both ends. I can barely walk, let alone hold that glass. My whole body aches, I have chills and I'm nauseous. I can't take another sip. I feel like I have the flu."

Jeff put his hand on my leg. "Should you call the doctor? Maybe you need to stop and do this when you feel better," he suggested.

"I can't stop now. I'm so close to getting an answer." I stopped in mid-thought, stared at Jeff, stone-faced, and took short breaths to fight the nausea. "I need help to the bathroom, quickly!" He flipped the comforter off me, lifted me up and helped move my feet to the floor.

"Can you walk?"

I nodded. He wrapped his arm around my back to support me as I moved to the bathroom. "Just lean on me. Do you have the runs or have to vomit?"

"Both."

He sat me down on the toilet and leaned the garbage pail on my lap so it was in front of my face. When I started to vomit, he held my hair back with one hand and rubbed my back with the other. My arms dangled and tears filled my eyes when I looked at him with the same expression Buddy gave us when he needed to go 'hurry ups.'

"You have to call the doctor. This is crazy."

Just then, the phone rang. "Are you ok if I answer the phone?" I nodded, then rested my head on the rim of the pail. It was my sister. Melissa was two and a half years older than me. As a teenager, I turned to her every time I got myself into trouble because she thought fast and had a way with words. She was the one who reasoned with my parents, hoping to soften each punishment.

Jeff described the situation and said I would call her back. "She agreed with me," he said. "This isn't normal and we should call the doctor."

I was grateful to get back into bed and left my number with the doctor's service. When the phone rang, Jeff placed it by my ear to update the doctor.

"I won't be able to treat you if you postpone," the doctor said. "I want to help you but you must finish the drink."

Jeff hung up, grabbed the glass and stuck the straw in my mouth until I finished the drink. He dimmed the bedroom lights on his way out. "Just holler if you need me." I nodded and focused on the chipped paint on our wall, feeling just as worn out.

Thirty minutes later, Abby peeked her face through the crack of my bedroom door. I forced a smile and spoke loud enough so that she could her me. "I see you, cutie."

She opened the door and walked towards the foot of my bed, smiling back. She was about to climb up with me and paused. "If I lie next to you, am I going to get what you have?" she asked, staring at my belly. It looked as if a basketball was hiding under the duvet cover.

"Of course not," I said, but the truth was that I had no idea. If I was right the first time, and this was giardia, then yes, she *could* get what I had, but no one had confirmed any diagnosis.

Abby was as uninformed as the rest of us, including the doctors. As much as I wanted her to move closer, I was nervous when she did. What if I passed this to her or anyone in our family? I did not want them to suffer or miss school or work.

Abby's courage astounded me. She lay down next to me, resting her head on one of my pillows. While she giggled and shared stories, I smiled and pretended to be interested, focusing on my severe stomach cramps. When the pain was unbearable, I managed to get out of bed and walk toward the bathroom, feeling Abby's eyes on me, wondering what was wrong. I imagined I looked like an old woman, creeping along.

"Just give me a sec," I mumbled and sat down on the bathroom floor. I leaned my head on the rim of the toilet seat to vomit. By the time I left the bathroom, Abby was gone.

I underwent the colonoscopy the next morning. When I woke up in the outpatient recovery unit, I heard my doctor's voice. "Everything looks good. No infections. Your colon is clear. I would suggest you eat more roughage."

That was all he had to say? *Eat more roughage?* I wasn't sure I heard him correctly, being so groggy after the procedure. I glanced at Jeff.

"That's all she eats," he said. "Isn't there anything else she can do?"

I stared at the doctor, hoping he had more to offer.

"I should have your blood work back tomorrow," the doctor said. "Let's see what comes from that. When you're ready, get dressed."

Jeff helped me change into my sweats and walked me to the car. At the first traffic light, he tried to comfort me, placing his hand on my thigh. No matter how much he wanted to help me, I was too angry to be comforted then. I could not believe that all of this came down to eating more fiber and leafy green foods. Worse, I was frustrated that the doctor had dismissed all other possibilities and I refused to believe his explanation was correct. When the light turned green, I pulled my leg away from Jeff and faced the window, remaining silent the whole ride home. Though Jeff was obviously doing everything he could to support me, I felt alone and terrified.

I found refuge on our hunter green couch, my favorite spot when I wasn't in bed. Jeff asked, "Can I get you something before I leave for work?" I shook my head. "Did you call your mother? You know she's waiting by the phone for the results." I shook my head again.

"Are you ok?"

I shrugged.

"I know you're disappointed that we didn't get answers. Maybe the blood work will show hypothyroidism. At least nothing is seriously wrong."

I wanted to believe him and glanced down at my belly. I covered my legs with the throw blanket, hearing Buddy's collar jiggle when he trotted in from the kitchen. He placed his snout on my lap, nudging my knees until I petted his head. I looked backed at Jeff.

"Can you just call and tell her?" I couldn't face discussing any of this without answers. All I wanted to do was rest and watch television until the girls got home from school.

CHAPTER
9

I LOOKED FORWARD to a "week of nothing" during winter break; however, on the first day, I wanted to attend the funeral of a pre-school colleague. Many people in the community were devastated by her sudden heart attack at the beginning of the week, during school hours. I just so happened to be in the play area, down the hall from the music room where she collapsed. I saw teachers and the nurse running with the defibrillator. I had been haunted ever since.

My mind leapt to conclusions. As I waited in bed while Jeff showered, I wondered if I would be the next to die. My illness had only gotten worse. How much more sickness could my body handle?

"Your turn!" he said when he finished, but I could not move. His words struck a nerve. It was not my turn—to die. I thought of Abby, Jolie. My family. My friends. As Jeff approached the bed,

I wiped my tears on the sheets and felt another searing pain in my stomach. I groaned.

"You'll feel better if you take a hot shower," he offered among several suggestions. Lately, showers were spent staring down at my feet, watching more strands of hair clog the drain. How could that help? Although today, my hair was the least of my concerns. I shot down every one of his ideas until he had nothing left to offer.

"I'll wake the girls and get them situated in the kitchen before I leave for work."

I refused to let him go.

I sighed. "I can't skip the funeral but it feels like someone's hands are inside my stomach, ripping through my skin."

He looked at me in disbelief. "Skip the funeral and still take the girls to their play dates. I'm sure their friends' mothers would understand. Everyone knows how sick you've been. Just call and ask if they would watch them a little longer today." He rushed to get dressed. When he left the bedroom, he kissed my forehead to say goodbye. "Let me know what you decide to do."

I reached for the phone on my nightstand and called a friend who I planned to carpool with to the funeral. I explained my situation, and then managed to get out of bed. I took my black sweatpants from the floor, lifting each leg ever so slightly into them, worried I would set off more shooting pains through my belly. I kept on the same red tanktop on that I had slept in and walked into the kitchen, hunched over in a ninety-degree angle. My girls waited at the table for breakfast. They knew I was not well today.

"What do you girls want to eat?"

"Pancakes, but why are you standing like that?" Jolie asked, squinting and fussing with her napkin.

I glanced at Abby because she didn't respond. She just stared back at me.

"I'm fine girls. It's just from some cramping in my stomach, but I'll be fine." I opened the freezer, grabbed the pancakes and placed them in the toaster. I held onto the countertop, taking slow, short breaths and waited for the toaster to buzz—ending the long silence.

"I'm still playing at Lucienne's house today right? You're not canceling it?" Abby asked.

Jolie added, "Me too. I'm supposed to go to Ashley's. You told me last night."

I took a deep breath and clenched my jaw as I reached for two plates in the cabinet.

"You're both going to your friends' homes to play. I'm just going to rest while you're out." I knew it was hard on them when I continuously changed their plans.

Once I gave the girls their Aunt Jemima pancakes and glasses of organic skim milk, I sat down at the table. I propped my head up with my hand and feigned interest in their conversation.

Jolie's forehead creased as she commented, "There's no syrup on the table."

I shut my eyes in agony, knowing I was the one who provided all that they needed during meals and begged, "Oh, Jo, please this time get it yourself."

She sighed and got up from the table, mumbling on her way to the cabinet, "Other moms get it for their kids but because you're always sick and tired, we do everything now. It's not fair."

I felt a large lump in the back of my throat, looking at Abby to see if she agreed. It was clear she empathized with her sister. Tears rolled down my cheeks.

I could barely get the words out. "I'm sorry, girls. I'm trying to get better."

When they finished eating, I asked them to get dressed, picking their own clothes. I used to love helping them with this, but was too tired and needed to rest in bed while they got ready. I needed some sympathy and dialed my mother, recalling a childhood wounding. She had become my confidante after I sat down at therapy with her to free myself from years of heartache.

A week before I had started Kindergarten, I played on the monkey bars at my neighbor's house and slipped and fell on my wrist. It was the first time I felt intense pain and ran straight home, holding my arm tight against my waist. I held back the tears until my mom opened our front door and saw my discomfort. Thirty-one years later, and I felt like that six year old again.

I weeped. "I am in so much pain I can barely move. I feel like I have aliens inside my stomach."

"When did that start? Aren't you going to the funeral this morning?" she asked.

"I canceled. Once the girls get dressed, I'm supposed to drive them to their friends' homes and come back to rest."

"Okay, but why the pain?"

Trying to relieve the last wave of pain, I slowly turned on my side in fetal position. I took a quick breath before I answered. "I don't know, but I can't take it and don't know if any rest will make it go away."

"I feel terrible about being so many miles away," my mom said from Lancaster, Pennsylvania, almost three hours from my sister and me in New Jersey. "I can't do anything from here."

"That's not the point. Just tell me what to do. I need help," I pleaded.

She heard the desperation in my voice and took command, like any mother with a sick child. "Listen to me, carefully. You are going to drop the girls off at their play dates and drive directly to the emergency room. Call Jeff, have him meet you there and make sure he calls me once a doctor gives you some idea of what is going on."

I wiped my tears on the pillowcase and hesitated. "I don't think I can drive. I'm really in bad shape."

"You can and you will. Get up, go and call me as soon as you know something. I love you very much. Now go."

I managed to get in the car and drive us safely to the first house to drop off Abby. When I pulled into her friend's driveway ten minutes from our home, she asked, "Could you walk me to the front door because I don't want to go alone?"

My body hurt too much to move an inch. I closed my eyes for a moment, feeling that same lump in the back of my throat, knowing it reappeared every time I said no to the girls' requests.

As I unlocked the car door, I experienced another shooting pain inside my abdomen and winced. "Come on Abby, really? You're a big girl. Just go, you'll be fine, I promise," I said, realizing my tone was a little too harsh.

She begged, "Please come with me, mommy."

I slowly inhaled and calmly continued. "I can see you from here." Even though I heard the whimpering in her voice, I couldn't find the strength to move and I needed help of my own. I sighed. "Just get a grip, Abby. It's fine!"

Jolie stepped up. "I'll walk you to the door, Ab."

With blurry eyes, I looked through the rearview mirror and hoped to get Jolie's attention in order to thank her, but they got out of the car too fast.

When Jolie hopped back in the car, she looked out the side window and shared, "She's fine." The rest of the drive, she sat in silence. This was not typical for Jolie. Usually, she told me long-winded stories or asked me tons of questions. Not today. My heart felt a heaviness that seemed to be the norm these days.

In order to hold back my tears, I didn't speak either. Five minutes later, I pulled into Ashley's driveway. As I placed the car in park and the doors automatically unlocked, Jolie pushed open the door and darted out. She shouted, "Feel better, mom," and never looked back.

By the time I lowered the window and hollered "I love you," she was at the front door and had not heard me. The scant time I had with my girls was filling with disappointments. I managed a half smile when Ashley's mom waved after Jolie walked inside.

The wait in the ER was all too familiar between the cubicle, background noises and scans. I called the mothers of both my daughter's friends and they agreed to watch them longer, promising to keep my situation to themselves. Two hours later, Jeff showed up and kissed my forehead. He seemed a bit frazzled.

"Sorry, I had to make sure my guys were set before I left the office."

I gave him a brief update and told him I was up next to go for scans. When I returned, I found Jeff watching ESPN News, sitting back on the familiar bedside chair, TV remote in hand, feet propped on my gurney. He asked me the routine questions and I responded with one-word answers, mostly avoiding eye contact. He mistook my frustration for anger towards him, which seemed to be typical for us lately. The longer the distance between a correct diagnosis, the greater the silence we shared. I did not like this space any more than he did. We were both terrified but too afraid to admit how much we'd lose if the diagnosis proved to be incurable.

He handed me the endocrinologist's name and number that he got from my sister, while the on-call doctor at the hospital reiterated old news: the severe pain in my abdomen was a result of backed up stools. "Unfortunately, we can only relieve the constipation but not alleviate the acute problem at hand, which is probably what is causing the repetitive ER visits," he said.

He wrote me some prescriptions while a nurse arrived with a laxative and paperwork. I was too familiar with the routine. "I would suggest you make an appointment with a gastroenterologist to work on solving the underlying problem," he said.

I returned home later that night, ten hours after disappointing my children. While Jeff picked up the girls from their play dates, I walked through the kitchen and noticed Buddy standing next to our sliding doors, scratching the glass with his paw, but instead of relieving him, I turned away and continued towards the bedroom. Though I felt badly about ignoring his needs, I only wanted to escape, and confront my own. I got into bed, turned on the television and raised the volume to drown out Buddy's whimpers. Golden Retrievers are known to please their masters, and Buddy waited until Jeff got home to relieve himself.

CHAPTER
10

J ANUARY 2009 STARTED with high hopes, only to be destroyed by doctor consultations. First, I met with an endocrinologist through my sister's contact. Lately, it took an enormous amount of effort to get myself to and from these appointments. The energy involved in showering, clothing and getting the girls off to school felt like I had just finished another half-marathon. I could not believe how little I could do with the weakness and bloating. At least losing my hair prevented me from putting any effort into blow-drying it.

The endocrinologist told me that my blood work showed low thyroid levels. My thyroid stimulating hormone, known as TSH, was normal so the results from the blood work didn't prove a clear-cut case of hypothyroidism. He prescribed Synthroid, to raise the T4 levels, and Cytomel for the T3 levels, hoping both would jump-start my metabolism. While I started the medication, I consulted with a second gastroenterologist, convinced I was suffering from more than low thyroid levels.

I seized the first available appointment at 7:30 in the morning, yet another major inconvenience for my family, requiring me to wake the girls early and bring them along before school started while I filled out more paperwork. They were not thrilled to be left in an empty waiting room, watched by nurses they never met while they ate breakfast in silence. It was another reminder that life was now about "mommy's illness."

When my examination was over, the doctor read through what had become my portfolio of past appointments and scans. He was eager to diagnose my condition. He scheduled an endoscopy a few days later. I tried to be thorough while I had the doctor's undivided attention, but rushed through the appointment, guilt-ridden over leaving my children behind. I longed for the days when carpools, play dates and math homework were my biggest dilemmas. When I handed my credit card to the nurse, I remembered a key question. Luckily, the doctor still stood ten feet from me. "Wait, what about the parasite my dog had this past summer, giardia, could I have that?" I asked, realizing I had stopped telling people this information. I could see Jolie rolling her eyes, annoyed that I prolonged our departure. She was only in second grade, how much more patience could I expect? I reached for her hand, gently rubbing my thumb over her knuckles. I tried to tend to her needs, even if it was only a small gesture.

The doctor concluded that my symptoms didn't match up with a parasite, and that giardia was highly unlikely. "That's why I have you doing the take home stool tests anyway," he said, reassuring me. "I'll see you in a few days at the endoscopy. We'll get you better."

Later, I told Jeff, "I like this doctor, I feel like he's going to figure it out."

I woke from the endoscopy to learn that everything looked normal. I should've been elated to hear this news. Instead, I was very frustrated. I was feeling anything but normal.

The doctor left the recovery room to write a prescription and a nurse placed her hand on my shoulder. "Don't look so disappointed. That's a good thing. You don't want the doctor to find anything."

I couldn't disagree more. I wanted the doctor to find something—anything to make sense of my situation. "Why do I still feel and look this way?" I mumbled, glancing towards my belly.

The nurse said nothing and patted my wrist, then smiled before leaving the room.

The doctor returned with a prescription called Amitzia. I was to take one pill, three times per day with my meals. "This should relieve the bloat and the constipation as it helps with intestinal mobility. I'll call you when the results to your stool sample come back."

I finished another outpatient procedure feeling weak, bloated, and now gassy. I sat up on the gurney, my bare legs dangling below, and stared at my clothes, trying to hold back tears. A part of me actually considered wearing the oversized hospital gown home, instead of squeezing back into my sweats and being reminded of my mysterious distended belly and weight gain.

The knock at the door startled me. "Trace, do you need any help?" Jeff asked.

I looked down at my clothes that were still folded. "I'm almost done. I need a few minutes. Just wait there," I said loud enough, knowing I needed space. Lately, his pep talks only caused me to withdraw even further.

The doctor's office called later that week. "The stool samples were clean. Just continue taking Amitzia and follow up in a month." I wasn't willing to wait this time.

❖ ❖

Over the next month, between the girls' school hours and my doctor visits, I dragged myself back to the gym despite feeling like a pile of cement. I sat in my car on the phone with either my mother or therapist, whoever was available at the time, agonizing over this harsh new reality; nothing had changed. I only seemed to be getting worse.

I hardly mustered the energy to step on the gas pedal, let alone walk through the parking lot at the gym. I kept my head down inside, passing the many mirrored walls. I didn't recognize myself and I avoided any false reflections I perceived of my body.

This so-called sickness exposed character flaws I didn't want to face. With help from my therapist, I was able to see that much of my self-worth was based on how I looked. It was clear that most of my insecurities originated from my need to have things be "perfect." I wasn't sure what bothered me more: the fact that I had no control over the changes of my body and hair, or that this horrible situation was happening to only me.

I barely completed fifteen minutes on an elliptical machine, while my friends continued their workouts with the stamina I once possessed. I was starting to sense that the bloat only worsened when I exercised. I should have stopped, but my mind was clouded with resentment.

Still, I was desperate to find a way back to the treadmills. While on the elliptical machine, I heard two friends trade stories about their recent appointments with an energy healer who also connected with "the other side." What that exactly meant, I wasn't quite sure.

Each friend testified how the healer addressed their past without knowing anything about them. I paused, considering the only "spiritual experience" I ever had was passing a blinking sign for a psychic reading on my way to work when I lived in New York City. There were millions of times I wanted to consult a psychic, but figured it was a load of crap and a waste of money. However, the great skeptic in me was fascinated by the possibility of a medium ever since a dear friend died in a car accident at the end of my freshman year of college. I was devastated that I missed his funeral because of a final exam, which left me without the opportunity to say goodbye. Now that I was at the end of my rope, I prayed an energy reading could diagnose and heal me. I got an appointment a week later.

I expected a dark room with crystal balls and incense, but the energy healer's office looked no different than what I'd seen at a massage therapist. Calming music played in the background. Diane, the healer, stood across the room, dressed in black Lycra leggings and a black tanktop which accentuated her red hair. She spewed a laundry list of health issues that matched every one of my symptoms. "Your hormones are out of whack. Your GI tract is off, your liver is clogged and your adrenals—oh, honey, your adrenal glands are hurting."

I stood motionless while she starred at me as if I had the plague.

"Does any of this make sense to you?"

I was stricken by her accuracy. "Yeah, definitely." This was the first medical intuitive I had ever met. She revealed private details of my friend Larry's car accident of which she had no way of knowing. Apparently, Larry's spirit was in the room and provided this information. Diane was even able to tell me what he looked like. She was totally accurate on that, too, but I couldn't help hear Jeff in the back of my mind, chuckling and rolling his eyes. *"Sometimes you're just so gullible. You're their perfect target."* Yet, everything Diane had said felt real. I kept my poker face contained, convinced that any facial expression could provide her with more clues.

She continued, "You're in the forest, on your knees crying and about to give up. Don't. You are almost there—to the other side, you'll see the light soon. You must keep going. This experience is the metamorphosis of your soul and you will one day write a book about your life lessons. You will help so many others heal. You are not alone."

My mouth opened in shock. My eyes welled up. It felt as if she spoke to my soul.

"How did you know that?"

I wondered if Diane read minds since I never shared any vision of my future, not even to my mother. At the end of our one-hour session, she insisted I meet Chris Butler, a holistic acupuncturist who specialized in women's herbal medicine.

I had never considered using new age healers. I had never touched herbal medicine or done acupuncture. The image of needles sticking out of my skin left me uneasy and suspicious, but I was so desperate that I was willing to see Chris as a last resort. Diane believed he would change my life, and I made an appointment the next day without even checking a reference.

Chris worked in a small, unimpressive office in a town twenty minutes from where I lived. He was in his early fifties, wore preppy glasses and dressed right from a Brooks Brothers catalog. During our consultation, he reviewed my records and spent quality time with me. He introduced a different perspective I had never heard of before called functional medicine, which starts with the premise that the human body is a functional whole. He explained how the body's organ systems inte act and penetrate on the most minute levels, so when one system breaks down, it affects the function of the other systems, causing a domino effect that can take place over a short or extended period of time.

He was honest and forthright in sharing his version of my downfall. "Adrenal glands provide a spark-plug effect to the mitochondria. They are energy factories of our body. When there are problems with the blood sugar, inflammation or even adrenal or thyroid glands, the mitochondrial function is impaired and a person feels fatigued or wiped out. Over time, these systems under-function and the situation becomes serious," he said, revealing the effects that daily behaviors have on the body.

The infertility medication, over-exercising and yo-yo dieting topped the list of my demise. In past years, I used food as a way to numb my feelings. Even though I knew eating unhealthy would eventually harm my body, I only cared about my physique. Five months before the half marathon, I became a conscious eater to be in ultimate shape. I cut any products containing sugar and white flour from my diet. After hearing Chris' concerns, I was relieved my diet was consistent with his recommendations.

He mentioned how the body knows what it needs by something called the hypothalamus-pituitary-adrenal axis—the feedback loop that continuously sends cellular messages from the pituitary gland to other systems such as the thyroid and adrenal glands. He offered to help rebalance my systems through acupuncture and herbal supplements.

"Acupuncture helps reroute the blocked pathways caused by inflammation on a cellular level while the supplements support and rebuild the immune system. If you follow my regimen, I think I can help you feel better." I'd try anything at this point.

I left his office with a bag full of supplements, a months' worth of scheduled appointments and a hard pitch to sell Jeff on this idea.

I sat alone at the kitchen table in a daze with my hands holding up my head when Jeff got home from work. "What are all those bottles on the counter? There are so many."

I flinched and prepared my speech. "I had a consultation with that acupuncturist today."

Jeff rolled his eyes while he skimmed through the mail. I

continued, "Actually, this was the first time anyone explained what's happening to my body and it made some sense."

I slowly stood, resembling someone in their eighties and leaned against the granite, standing next to the numerous bottles of supplements.

He put the mail down and turned to me, unimpressed. "So what did he say?"

I took a deep breath. "Apparently, my adrenal glands are spent from years of stress I placed on them. So, all the infertility treatments, severe exercise regimens and unhealthy eating habits in past years contributed to it."

I knew from the look on Jeff's face, I wasn't pleading my case very well. I should have tape recorded the appointment and replayed what transpired because I knew there was no way I could reiterate Chris's explanations, but I tried anyway.

Jeff stared at me in disbelief.

"He thinks he could help and get me back on track. I just have to do acupuncture twice a week and take those supplements for a while."

Jeff shook his head in frustration. "How much is all that going to cost? I bet none of it's covered by our insurance, right? Did you happen to notice the bills that we're getting from your other consultations and hospital visits? Those are piling up too, Trace."

I crossed my arms, knowing this discussion wasn't going to end very well.

"What do you want me to do, Jeff? Live this way? Do you have another solution? Because I sure don't." I walked back to the kitchen table, plopped down on my seat and beckoned the girls with whatever energy was left, "Girls, dinner's on the table."

Without waiting for anyone else, I grabbed my fork and stared down at my plate of quinoa and sautéed kale. Jeff and

I didn't say a word to each other during dinner and I refused to look at him. When I made conversation, it was directed only towards the girls. He tried to break the tension between us, when he purposely asked for the one dressing that only I could reach. I ignored him more than once without it being blatantly obvious to the girls.

"It's fine, don't worry. I don't need any dressing on my salad. Lettuce is great when it's plain," he joked, assuming I'd break into laughter. I refused to end my silent treatment or give him the satisfaction of seeing his infamous smart-ass smirk.

When we had disagreements in the past, Jeff always found a way to end them with some sort of sarcastic joke. His sense of humor was one of the things I loved most about him as it helped to ease my intensity. In our relationship, he was the one who lightened our serious conversations and the toughest moments between us. It was because of him that I survived the years of infertility treatments and rocky pregnancy. When I was sick, he took care of me, even if it meant he missed out on times with his buddies, whether on the golf course, basketball court or a night out watching a sports game. He kept his head held high, rarely complained and was easy to please. He accepted people and his situations as they were, without judgment. Even if he felt stressed, Jeff never complained about carrying the weight.

My sickness was beginning to take a toll on him now. I didn't need a psychic to provide such insight. I was his wife and lived with him for more than ten years already. Of course I noticed his many grunts and scowls when he looked through the mail, listened to my daily complaints, and watched as I pulled away from him— especially in our bedroom. The more distance I put between us, the more I witnessed the change in his disposition.

At this point, there was no way to comfort me. I just wanted my life to go back to the way things were just before we got Buddy.

Nothing relieved my misery, regardless of Jeff's choice of comforting words. He could not provide the answers I needed then, which only compelled me to retreat further. I hated that my husband, my protector, the man I trusted most, couldn't find a way to fix me. What I hated even more was the realization that my sickness had hardened his personality. While he tried to seem upbeat coming home from work, I sensed defeat in his voice. He was fighting to keep his business alive while the economy tanked, trying to provide the comfortable life we once had while I continued to increase our expenses. He was getting pounded from every direction. The last thing he needed was his wife's bitterness and resentment when he walked in the door. On some occasions, when I was lying on the den couch, Jeff turned off his car and hung out in the garage for some time. I assumed he needed to be alone.

Despite his fears, I wished he didn't bring finances into our discussion. I needed him to have faith that acupuncture could work, regardless of the fact that neither of us understood it. The last thing I wanted to hear was Jeff's skepticism. I was determined to give Chris a chance.

After a few weeks of treatment, I noticed a difference in some symptoms. The severe pressure in my abdomen lessened a bit. Though I still experienced constipation, I was able to get relief much faster. Most significantly, I was amazed at the shift in my state of mind and how I was able to leave Chris's office after each session. He suggested I stop taking birth control pills and complete a take-home saliva test for a more accurate reading of my hormone levels. Miraculously, Jeff stopped arguing about the costs of these treatments, trying his hardest to be supportive, especially now that there was evidence that my symptoms were improving.

"I've had patients with blood work that states one thing but their saliva tests prove differently and you may fall under this category." He mentioned the possibility that too much estrogen or not enough testosterone could cause my symptoms to match up to someone with hypothyroidism, even when my blood results weren't consistent with those findings. He explained that taking certain prescribed medications masks the underlying issues, causes side effects and puts more stress on the liver.

I was never truly comfortable about my decision to start birth control after my college experience. "Honestly, I was pushed into taking the pill. Three different doctors agreed it was the only way and that I should be fine. Look at me now. There's got to be a connection between my hormones, the weight gain and severe fatigue, right?" I asked.

Chris never looked at his watch during our appointments. He gave me his undivided attention when we were together and provided explanations to all of my questions as thoroughly as possible. He spent extra time in order for me to understand how birth control pills worked within the body. Having these numerous heartfelt conversations with Chris, I took his advice and stopped the pills by February. I completed the saliva take-home test after I read the directions three times. I collected enough of my spit to fill six different vials every two hours for twelve hours. I froze the vials until the next day then Fed Ex'd the package to Geneva Laboratories and waited three weeks for results.

The more time I spent with Chris, the more detailed our conversations got. He appreciated all that I learned from Kathy's nutritional sessions regarding food options, but he also wanted to rule out any allergens that might be contributing to my inflammation. He confirmed that I had food sensitivities through more saliva tests, and suggested I cut all those foods from my diet.

This made zero sense.

"I never had to cut anything from my diet before other than to watch my weight. How is it possible I am allergic to so many foods now?" I asked.

He handed me the test results and I scanned through the list, wondering why gluten appeared when I had tested negative for Celiac's Disease by one of the gastroenterologists. Soy and dairy were also on the list. My spirit sank when I saw eggs.

"Oh my god! I can't have eggs, not even egg whites? I live on egg whites!"

Chris saw my frustration and placed my file on the table. He explained to me how the test is broken down by the level of severity each food has on the immune system. For example, pinto, kidney or navy beans were towards the bottom of the list and in the first bracket. Translation: my body may or may not react to them and if it did, it wouldn't be too severe.

I rolled my eyes, wishing that were the case with eggs. I didn't eat those kinds of beans. He continued and pointed towards the top of the list explaining that gluten, soy, dairy, peanuts and even eggs may be too hard on my body to digest and could cause severe symptoms like headaches, constipation, fatigue and bloat. That made sense, but didn't leave me with much to eat. I had already cut out sugar, white flour and coffee.

Now, I was to eat only plain fish or chicken for protein, brown rice, quinoa, millet and amaranth for carbohydrates, dark leafy greens for vegetables, fruits, and two tablespoons of either sunflower or pumpkin seeds, walnuts, almonds or almond butter for snacks. I could dress my salads with olive or flaxseed oil and lemons. I added up the minimal calories, unable to make sense of the progressive weight gain. "One thing at a time," he said gently, preparing for our acupuncture session. As he placed each needle on the specific pressure points, he was eager to hear of my next consultation with a new internist who specialized in functional medicine.

CHAPTER
11

Doctor Zacharias came with perks. His office was close to our house, and he was a primary care physician who practiced functional medicine and accepted my insurance, which Jeff appreciated. It was a comfort to know my therapist found an experienced doctor, one who had the qualifications to lead my case and help me heal. He had come highly recommended from her other patients.

"He listens to his patients, looks at the body as a whole and has terrific bedside manners. I think this could be a great match," my therapist said. I was eager since I placed zero effort in finding a new internist.

I had driven past Dr. Zacharias' office building many times but never knew this would become my new second home. He shared his office space with a dentist and didn't have a receptionist. Instead, he appeared in the doorway on time with my folder full of records. He was of average height, slender, sported gray hair and a matching beard, styled like something in GQ.

"Tracey Berkowitz," he stated with exuberant charm. I was the only patient in the waiting room. He continued, "Come on in!"

I followed him to his office and sat down, lugging the heavy weight from my slow body. As I reviewed the sequence of events that led me to this visit, I found something oddly familiar about him. Our conversation flowed during his examination. I never sat in silence, unlike the many doctors I had seen. He asked various questions about my family, lifestyle and even covered conversations from past appointments with other doctors. He cracked jokes every chance he got to lighten my mood.

We headed into his examination room. He asked me to run through my most recent symptoms as he drew my blood. "Or is that too much multi-tasking for you?" He winked. I chuckled, appreciating his sense of humor.

"My body feels like cement. I sleep all the time and have severe constipation. My hair is falling out in the shower or when I slide my fingers through it, and I gained fifteen pounds, so I stopped weighing myself. I can't bear to look at the number rise anymore," I glanced down at my belly. "And because of all this inflammation, my acupuncturist has me avoiding many foods that are too sensitive for my immune system."

He finished the blood test and pulled the tourniquet off my arm.

"Look who's doing her homework," he said, validating every suggestion my acupuncturist had made. "Do you have any other symptoms?"

I nodded. "I get headaches sometimes and numbness in my toes. But out of all my issues, that's the least of my concern."

Before he weighed me, he asked, "Do you want to face the other direction or take it like a man?" I faced the numbers. I gained another five pounds, twenty in total. My shoulders slumped. It was another reminder that I wasn't imagining the weight gain.

He suggested a home stool test to check for giardia, among other parasites, then ordered a twenty-four hour urine collection to rule out mercury poisoning.

"Mercury poisoning? That's a first," I said, alarmed.

"You have some of the symptoms and you eat a lot of fish." He opened his drawer and pulled out a card that listed the fish carrying high levels of mercury, then told me to avoid eating the fish on the left side of the list for now. He noticed my hesitation.

"Does that leave you anything to eat?"

I shook my head. I had to eliminate two of my favorite fish, sea bass and tuna, which I ate at least once a week. He walked me to the reception area. "This is an easy case," he said and winked. "We'll figure it out. No worries, Berko!" I smiled, realizing I found my Doctor House.

Ten days later, I returned to Dr. Zacharias' office to review test results. He covered a list of topics, starting with my thyroid. The levels were still low, even with the two medications I was taking. He switched me to Armour Thyroid, an extract of the thyroid gland, which contains T4 and T3. Apparently, Armour Thyroid was the most natural medication and would have the least affect on the liver. He also suggested taking bio-identical hormone creams to help with my estrogen, testosterone and progesterone levels.

"The fatigue should get better as your hormone levels rise," he assured me.

The only thing I knew of bio-identical hormones I had heard from Suzanne Summers on Oprah. She looked vibrant.

"I'll try it," I said, relieved to hear that my stool test came back negative.

"No parasites. That's good," he said, "But your mercury levels are extremely high."

He recommended chelation therapy to treat acute mercury poisoning. To detoxify myself I would have to take four pills, three times per day for three days, then stop for three days and repeat that two week cycle for multiple rounds in order for my numbers to return to normal.

"You realize that means no more fish, Berko," he said, though I was very disappointed to hear that. "I think this is the underlying culprit causing your body havoc. We have some answers. That's good."

Mercury poisoning was a hard sell. When I shared my diagnosis with Jeff, my mother, a co-worker or friend, I constantly fumbled on words. It didn't matter who saw my belly, the response was always the same, "No way that's from mercury poisoning!"

Even I wasn't convinced, but I stopped at nothing to heal. I took large amounts of supplements and medication daily, and avoided most foods on the lists. My new way of life not only became second nature for me, but also for my family and friends. Instead of exercising, I spent my mornings sorting through bottles of pills and popping them in Ziploc bags, according to the time I needed to take them—with meals or on an empty stomach. I was as organized as any mother who left the house with a baby. My handbag turned into a diaper bag for the chronically ill.

Since I was already a finicky salad eater, my close friends were used to my way of ordering meals when I met them for lunch. If I forgot to take my pills on an empty stomach before I left the car, I'd take them in restaurants, which led to conversations about my health. Some friends listened to my explanations whether they understood or not, while others drilled me with more questions and hoped their recommended doctor would have better answers. They were as perplexed as I was that a lifestyle of healthy eating could cause such weight gain.

When I dressed up for my niece's Bat Mitzvah at the end of February, no magic wand could fix my perception of the pumpkin-like body I inhabited. I tried to put my obsession for a quick fix aside, and fought the fatigue in order to participate in my family's celebration. I even made an appointment to have my hair done, keeping my mind off of that issue. Although, it didn't help when my hairdresser held onto the sides of my hair while he stared at me through the mirror and commented, "The texture of your hair feels different. Have you noticed?" Ah, yeah. You think I haven't noticed?

I nodded, wincing that someone other than myself saw the difference in my hair. I wasn't imagining this and it wasn't just stress. I spent the rest of the time in his seat, wondering if a wig was in my future.

I borrowed a co-worker's dress for the Friday night service. It was a black, short-sleeved, a-lined sweater dress. The previous month, I bought two different dresses, both black to disguise my weight. By the time the Bat Mitzvah weekend arrived, I had gained more weight. The new dresses were already too tight, and the last place I wanted to stand was on the temple Bima, spotlighting my extra pounds.

While my family was getting dressed, I stood in the entryway of our house, panicked over what to wear to the party. Jeff shouted, "You look fine in the dress you're wearing. There's not a lot of time to start changing." Oh, if he only knew. He was 5'8 and 165 lbs. He never had to be concerned about his physique. Didn't he understand the calamity of a woman having a panic attack at the closet? I picked up the phone to call my friend, Wendy, hoping to get her sympathies. When she heard the panic in my voice, she sent over her husband, David, with one of her dresses.

David stood in the front door, teasing me for the production I had made until he saw the expression on my face. "Trace, I didn't realize…Hopefully this will make it better?" He held up Wendy's dress, a two-piece crinkled silver bustier top with matching skirt. I wondered if her outfit would hide my stomach more than the skintight black dress I was wearing.

My mother glanced down at her watch and grabbed my shoulders, "Everyone knows what hell you are going through. Keep the dress you have on. You look beautiful even with the weight gain. No one sees you the way you do, and tonight it's about Alix's accomplishments. You are lucky to be alive and experience this so get yourself together!" She was right. This wasn't about me. I had five minutes to compose myself while she waited with my father in their car. On the way to the club, I fidgeted with my dress, grateful the party room would be dark.

CHAPTER
12

I
N LATE MARCH, I completed two rounds of Chelation Therapy, which lowered my mercury levels, reaching the high end of normal range. Chris studied every blood test, hoping to find a missing link, while my energy peaked for a few weeks, but quickly subsided despite the supplements, medications and acupuncture treatments.

By the end of the month, my body drifted into a coma-like state during a ski trip in Aspen, Colorado. We transferred more of our credit card points for another set of free flights and stayed at a timeshare condominium, this time owned by Jeff's parents. I could barely walk, talk or even laugh. I remained seated most of the trip with my head propped in my hands. I wanted so badly to partake in the fun, but my body wouldn't allow it. Instead, I watched my daughters' disgruntled faces from the sidelines, feeling that same heaviness in my heart, imagining their life without me. Silently, I begged to get my life back.

A major snowstorm gave me more time to sleep on the last two days while Jeff entertained the girls. In the rare moments I was actually awake, I lay lifeless, questioning my body's weaknesses. It took every last bit of energy to raise my hand a few inches from the pillow—to prove to myself I hadn't yet died. I was tired of the hours I'd spent alone in bed over the past months and felt as though my spirit was dying a slow death.

Jeff tiptoed into the bedroom, afraid of waking me. I noticed the worried look on his face when he saw my pale complexion and frail body. "You have to call the doctor when you get home," he said. "Tell him you got worse. This is ridiculous already—you can't function anymore!" It relieved me to know that he could finally see how I had been feeling all along.

I got an appointment to see my primary care physician the following week. His responsiveness renewed my confidence that he genuinely cared about my case. He took my complaints seriously and listened thoroughly to every new symptom.

The morning I got dressed for my appointment, Jeff lingered in our bedroom, already late for work. Buddy rested on our decorative pillows. Regrettably, my relationship with Buddy was definitely declining. Though I never talked to Jeff about it, I knew Buddy sensed my resentment.

Jeff watched as I reached for my jeans off the dresser. I felt both of them staring as I slowly put each leg in its hole. These were the last pair of "fat" jeans I owned, and they had gotten extremely tight during vacation. I gripped the two belt buckle loops with each hand as I pulled them up. I knew this was going to be a battle, which was why I chose not to wash them.

I figured the worst case scenario, these jeans would be skin tight and left unbuttoned. When I got as far as my kneecaps and realized they weren't budging any further, my breath shortened. The harder I tried to pull, the more frustrated I got. This can't be happening, I thought. I had worn these jeans four days ago. There was no way my body had changed that much in such a short time. The panic ushered in a new terror: I no longer had control over the size of my body.

I mentally reviewed everything I ate over the past week. I hadn't binged on vacation. I had not sat around the ski slopes eating chili dogs and fries, or evenonce said, "I'm on vacation, I can let this slide." I adhered to the same strict diet I'd been following for months. The foods and portions would have kept any healthy person's weight intact but I wasn't healthy. I was obviously very sick and my body kept expanding. I was seconds from a meltdown.

I heard Jeff's voice from across the room. "Which jeans are those?"

I stood up, looked towards his direction. "Same as the ones I wore during vacation," I blurted between sobs. "They won't even go above my thighs anymore. It's only been four days Jeff—four freaking days!"

He shook his head in amazement, walked across the room and wrapped his arms around me. "I'm so sorry," he whispered in my ear and hugged me tight, while my arms dangled at his sides. After a moment of silence, he leaned back and started to wipe the tears from one of my cheeks. As soon as I felt his touch, I turned my head and backed away. My reactions became automatic at this point, avoiding any shred of intimacy between us. I grabbed my black gym pants off the dresser and sat down on the bed, swapping them for the jeans. I climbed back into bed, staring at the jeans I left on the floor. He continued, "You're seeing the doctor today so tell him about this. If he doesn't have answers then we find another doctor that will!"

Jeff was right, but nothing he said could make me feel better.

I calmed down and caught my breath, "I just wish I could unzip this fat suit." It was my prison and I was left without a key.

After Jeff left for work, I rested in bed for another half hour before my appointment and called my mom. Buddy approached the bed, nuzzled his snout in my face, looking for attention. I interrupted my mother, looked Buddy in the eyes and asked, "What? What do you want from me?" He tilted his head as his ears perked up, but I refused to pet him. I rolled over with my back to him, hoping my mother would raise my spirits instead.

I fought the fatigue and drove safely to Dr. Zacharias' appointment and wept after another examination, blood tests and recap of the jean dilemma. "It's been almost a year and I'm starting to lose it. My therapist thinks when the fatigue is heightened, I'm more depressed." I couldn't agree more. He handed me a tissue. I wiped my tears. "Help me, please!"

He suggested increasing the amounts of hormonal creams to help with my depression, fatigue, weight gain and libido loss. "Rest as much as you can. Now's the time to delegate—take more off your plate." I rolled my eyes and wondered if that included hosting this year's Passover Seder for both our families. I knew he was right but when I agreed to have this holiday, I saw it as another opportunity to prove I hadn't completely disappeared from my life. I had always been the one to run our household. Other than our finances, I organized everything else. Giving up that control was the last thing I wanted to do. The very thought terrified me because it meant surrendering to this condition; and if that happened, I wasn't sure I'd be able to recover from such a deep depression.

"Ask Jeff, your family and friends to pitch in," he said.

"Everyone's already helping out and next week's April Break so my girls will be home from school," I said, alluding to a different game plan. "I can't take much more of this." I wiped my eyes again, confounded that I had once run miles but could barely finish a conversation now.

He walked me to the reception area and smiled. "I'm not giving up on you, Berko! You're just trying to ruffle my feathers. We'll figure it out!" I needed that to be true.

My acupuncturist agreed with my primary care physician to delegate responsibilities in general but he wasn't on board with increasing my hormonal creams. "I've said this before, blood tests aren't a good reading of your hormone levels and I don't agree with using medication to force your body to produce more hormones. It's not natural. I've seen cases with hormones too high that match your same symptoms." Chris suggested I stop the creams altogether, considering they could mask the underlying problems or even make my situation worse.

I successfully entertained twenty people from our extended family for my first Passover Seder—feeling like a very good and dutiful Jewish wife. Whatever was lurking inside me, there was no way I could delegate this cultural obligation. The food was delicious, the table setting looked elegant, and my exhaustion and despair were neatly hidden behind my fake smile. I tried to keep up with the conversations, listening to my friends tell me how they spent the week with their kids. I had focused on resting and preparing for the holiday but refused to let the rest of the week slip away. My girls deserved some fun, and I didn't care if I had to push my body to give them that.

Ignoring the doctors' orders, we awoke early the next morning, drove to the Upper East Side of New York City, shopped at Lester's—my girls' favorite clothing store—lunched at Googie's Diner, ate dessert at Dylan's Candy Bar and finished with Miley

Cyrus' new movie on opening day. I promised the girls we'd do it all. There was no way I was about to let them down again.

While we watched the previews, I was hit with a severe wave of exhaustion. This was the first opportunity I had to sit during the past two days. I glanced at my belly, horrified to see it had blown up even more. Though Chris's voice ran through my head, *"that's inflammation,"* I resorted to my old worn tapes, counting calories to see if I had maxed out my daily intake, unaware that this habit had turned into a debilitating obsession. I craved what most fashion magazines and the media sold—the perfect body image. I knew it was all a façade, but it was an illusion I chose to believe. There I was in a New York City movie theater with my daughters, counting calories instead of enjoying the show. How much more of my life would I miss because I was not paying attention to what mattered most?

When April break was over, the girls went back to school and I planted myself on the den couch. I needed a break from the bedroom. Most days the girls fended for themselves and looked forward to the evenings when Jeff got home. I learned how to delegate rather quickly for play dates and carpools. Jolie jumped at the chance to play at another house, ride with a different family, or anything to avoid what was happening before her eyes. She didn't appreciate the fact that I slept most afternoons. I overheard her conversation one day with a friend as they came upstairs from the basement, while I lay sprawled like a drunk on the couch.

"What's wrong with your mom," their friend asked, "Is she sick?"

"She's always like that," Jolie said. She internalized everything and lately, the last topic she wanted to discuss was my sickness.

Abby added, "Let's just get our own snacks. It's fine."

I tried to interject but had no strength. I wished our trip to the city stayed fresh in their minds. Here I was, cognizant of their conversation, yet I couldn't even respond to a single word my kids said. Is this what patients that are in a coma go through, listening to their loved ones praying and speaking, without being able to reply? It was hard enough saying no to all the physical activity I couldn't do with them. Had I now failed my daughters on some emotional level? All my best memories of caring for my girls throughout the years were erased by Jolie's four simple words. *She's always like that.* Couldn't she see that I was desperately digging my way out of this dark hole? I was doing everything I could to be anything but *like that.*

Jolie headed toward the kitchen sliding doors and shouted, "Aw Boo, have you been waiting there the whole time? Do you have to go hurry ups?" I heard the door open and shut a moment later.

When the girls were done with their snacks, I listened to their footsteps as they headed back to the basement. "I'll be one second guys," Abby said. I felt a tap on my back and heard her voice. "Mom, you need something? You ok?"

I tried to talk but grunted. At thirty-seven years old, I wondered if I was having a stroke, but as I lay there unable to speak, I panicked. No matter how hard I tried, I could not speak or move, though my mind was aware something was very wrong. These trances happened most afternoons only when my girls were home. Otherwise, when they were gone, I experienced complete blackouts.

CHAPTER
13

O VER THE NEXT FEW WEEKS in May 2009, I continued to search for a diagnosis and an open-minded gynecologist who believed in functional medicine. I received many recommendations but none matched until I bumped into my friend Dana, an assistant teacher who used to work at the same preschool that my girls had attended. When they were toddlers, Dana had held Abby in her arms after her elbows had been pulled out of their sockets. I remember rushing to the school and seeing her arms dangling while she sucked on an ice pop, which Dana held up to her mouth. I expected to find my daughter frightened and in tears, but she was giggling and enjoyed Dana's attention as if nothing was wrong. When I told Jolie she and her sister had to leave camp early, she cried. These were the hardest moments of raising twins. Dana offered her assistance and walked us all to my car. She had terrific instincts and I valued her opinion, but more than that, she owned a Golden Retriever a few years older than Buddy.

She invited me to Riker Hill Park after I dropped the kids off at school.

"Buddy will love it," she said. "There are three other Golden Retrievers and trust me, he'll sleep like a champ for the remainder of the day so you can rest." The only form of exercise Buddy was getting was a walk with Jeff after work; otherwise, he stayed inside the house with me or roamed the backyard. I joined Dana the next day and reluctantly took Buddy of the leash.

"He'll be fine," Dana said, and stared at me quizzically. "But will you? What exactly is wrong with you?"

I wasn't offended. She had every right to ask. My distended belly wasn't exactly easy to hide. I shared my story, gesticulating wildly, at how I needed to find a new gynecologist.

"I have the perfect doctor for you," she said, tossing a tennis ball to our dogs. Her sister had a tumor in her pituitary gland, completely messing up her endocrine system until she found a mother/daughter practice in the city. "You need to contact the daughter of the practice," she said and got me the number from her sister. I left the park with an exhausted dog and the last shred of hope I had for a truly new year: I made an appointment in late May, four days after my birthday.

It was May 22nd and the last thing on my mind was celebrating my 37th birthday, though I appreciated the fuss my friends were making and agreed to meet them for lunch. When I woke that morning, I noticed the bloat was the worst it had ever been and I was extremely fatigued.

I managed to get out of bed and stood naked in front of the full-length mirror, examining my belly. I could hold it in my hands like a pregnant woman in her ninth month, and I wondered if the new supplements or raising the levels of hormonal creams had triggered this recent episode. Even though I had only turned a year older, I felt like I had aged fifty years.

Later that morning, I opened the kitchen door and shouted, "Inside Bud!" I glanced at the clock and realized I was late to my acupuncture appointment with Chris.

Buddy didn't budge an inch. He waited on our lawn for my next command.

Leaning against the frame of the sliding glass doors, I said, "I have no patience for this game today. Come on Bud, inside!" Still, no movement.

I grabbed one of his favorite treats from Trader Joe's and waved it in my hand for him to see. "You want this? Come here!"

He got as close to the steps of our deck and stopped. I stamped my foot. "I don't have the strength for this! Come on," I said, then mumbled, "You dumb dog."

I tried to reason with him. "I'm counting to three and if you don't come inside, I'm closing the door!" He blinked and stared me down, so I left him outside, shut the door, and took a shower, dreading the simplest tasks in my own routine.

I didn't know what to wear on my birthday and stared into my closet with frustration, ruling out black sweatpants. I only had five options that fit. I chose my a-line shaped, orange floral sundress that I recently bought. I threw a beige stretch tanktop underneath, which covered three quarters of my belly and stepped into a pair of gold gladiator styled sandals. I even blew my hair straight despite another clump that fell out. As I walked through the kitchen, I found Buddy waiting outside by the door and I let him in, feeling guilty he had to wait for me. "Sorry Boo, but now I have to leave." I put him behind the kitchen gate and left the house.

When I pulled up to Chris' office, my cell phone rang. It was Dr. Zacharias.

"Hey Berko, how are you feeling this morning?"

"Tired."

"More than usual?"

I was always tired and I wasn't sure why he was asking me this obvious question.

"Sort of the same," I added, "But while I have you on the phone, I woke up extremely bloated this morning. It's worse than ever—I look as if I'm about to go into labor."

He sympathized with me and sounded concerned.

"I got your recent blood test results and it seems your thyroid levels dropped. With the numbers here, you should feel weak, light headed and I'm even worried you could pass out."

I was grateful for the validation from the blood work. Finally, my test results were confirming how I actually felt. I needed some evidence that this was not psychosomatic.

"So I'm not crazy? I'm not making this up?" I asked.

"Of course not. It's true," he said, acknowledging that blood tests don't lie. I appreciated his attempts to make me laugh and lower my anxiety.

He insisted I drive straight to the pharmacy after I finish with Chris's appointment. He ordered a new prescription and wanted me to take half a pill immediately. "I raised the level of your Armour Thyroid to 120 milligrams. That should make a difference and provide you with a boost in energy if you took a pill this morning. It should taper off by the end of the day. However, if you feel your heart racing or your hands shaking, call me right away."

I agreed to keep him posted and walked into Chris's office.

When I got his attention, I said, "Are you ready for this?" I stood at the reception desk and pulled my dress tight around my abdomen. His mouth dropped open.

"Oh god! When did that happen?"

"I woke up like this." From the look on his face, I wondered if I qualified for the Guinness Book of World Records. I repeated the conversation I just had with my primary care physician and handed over my Blackberry so he could see the blood results.

He looked up at me. "Are you eating any fats in your diet?"

"Exactly what Kathy and you told me to eat. Why?" I was eager to hear his response.

"Your triglycerides are extremely low which means your body is not absorbing any fats."

I wondered if that's why I had found a bud, leaf and partial stem of broccoli rabe in my stool, the same condition it entered—in one piece, even after I had chewed and swallowed. "I don't get it."

I incorporated a lot of fats into my diet: pumpkin and sunflower seeds, walnuts, almonds, almond butter in addition to olive and flaxseed oils. When I told Chris, he shook his head in disbelief and asked me to forward the blood results so he could review them in further detail. He reiterated the importance of communicating with my internist in case I felt like I was on speed.

Great, I thought. Just what I needed. Speed? I hadn't felt anything moving fast recently.

"Don't mess around with the thyroid medication, and stop the bio-identical hormones," he admonished, preparing needles for my acupuncture treatment. He shared a few stories of patients who had complications taking hormones and reminded me it could take up to ninety days for the hormones to leave my body. I appreciated his concern and trusted he would not give up on my case.

"I am done with hormones of any kind, except for thyroid medication," I promised, wondering if my new gynecologist would agree.

I drove immediately to the pharmacy, and following Dr. Zacharias' directions, took only half a pill more of my thyroid medication, relieved to no longer put other hormones in my body. By the time I met my friends for lunch, I felt jacked up on adrenaline. I didn't have to fake a smile. I felt as if that tiny pill had given me back some of my missing vitality. Bring on the speed! I felt great. I was greeted with many hugs, kisses and laughter as we joked about my upcoming due date and the sex of my unknown baby. Some even asked to touch my belly, amazed by the mysterious bloat.

They wanted updates but my news flashes only seemed to confuse them. I had a team of doctors that nobody, including myself, could keep straight: Kathy, my life coach/holistic nutritionist, a former gynecologist and primary care physician, two reproductive gynecologists, two gastroenterologists, an endocrinologist, Chris my acupuncturist, Dr. Zacharias, my current primary care physician and the most recent gynecologist I had yet to meet. They were baffled by my unexplained symptoms, but listened intently. I was overwhelmed by their acceptance and steadfastness; however, I felt my heart beating a mile a minute. I looked down at my hands and spread my fingers apart. It was such a relief to be able to move my body parts so easily even if I found them shaking. I wasn't concerned—yet.

My close friend, Rachel noticed I was distracted. She turned to me and quietly asked, "Are you ok?"

I nodded. "Yep." I didn't want this energized feeling to stop, especially on my birthday. I kept this secret to myself for another few minutes, replaying the warning from both Chris and my internist. I finally tapped her hand and whispered, "I'm kind of freaking out. My heart is racing and look at my hands." I spread my fingers apart for her to witness.

"Call the doctor," she said.

"I will when I leave here."

She changed the subject and shared a cute story about one of her three boys. I appreciated her ease, calmed down and joined the rest of the conversation.

When I got back to the car, I contemplated calling my internist. I knew this adrenaline high would fade by the end of the day, and decided against stopping it too soon. I wanted my family to experience the old me, even if only for a few hours before I turned back into a zombie.

CHAPTER
14

A COUPLE DAYS LATER, I actually believed I could drive in this altered state. Jolie's afternoon art class was twenty minutes from our house. I insisted she go since she already missed a few classes and the session was paid. While driving on the highway, I felt my eyelids grow heavy in the sunlight. I blinked, desperate to stay awake. When my head jerked, I knew I was in trouble. I opened the car windows and turned up the music, hoping to keep my eyes from closing again. I looked in the rearview mirror, worried my girls suspected something was wrong. Luckily they played their video games, oblivious to my fatigue. I was eager to reach the exit. When I got to the art class, the girls ran inside while I called my mother, hoping for another way home.

Hunched over, I leaned my head against the steering wheel. "Mom, I seriously could have killed them!" I tried to catch my breath while I wiped away my tears.

"You didn't and they are safe but you can't drive when you're too tired."

I interrupted. "But I'm always tired. Don't you know? This is who I am now!"

I lifted my head and leaned my elbow on the door as I wiped more tears. Was I supposed to blow off my kids' schedule just because I felt tired? For some time now, that was a daily occurrence for me and I hated knowing my girls roamed the house while I lay in bed with the door closed. They were seven years old with practically no supervision, and they were expected to take care of Buddy. The guilt I felt around all of this lessened only when they were at their friends' houses. I stopped having play dates at our house unless it was the weekend when Jeff could watch them. I often wondered if they were safer with their friends' parents than with me.

Sure, I was sick and my condition left me in awful shape, but no doctor had given me a death sentence. I felt I hadn't "earned the right" to waste all this time in bed. I was distraught over the person I had become and embarrassed by my lack of parental guidance. I had no faith in my skills as a mom anymore and even toyed with the idea of hiring some help. Other than having a baby nurse when the girls were born to show me the ropes, I did everything with them. I could multi-task as good as any, feeding one a bottle while burping the other over my shoulder, and holding conversations with friends. At age two, the girls and I had the stomach virus within hours of each other. We took turns puking in the toilet during the middle of the night, and as weak as I was, I could still comfort them.

Raising twins was my first priority and I was damn good at it until now. I was in a bad place to even consider the idea of getting help as an option—and to actually believe that help was a sign of weakness at all. The only thing clear to me then was the inevitable discussion I was avoiding with Jeff about our finances because I was draining every resource. I didn't want to end my marriage because I had asked for childcare, or worse, lose my husband's respect for me as a mother.

My mother's optimism quickly shifted my attitude, pervading all our phone calls.

"I believe this will all end soon. Until then, stop driving when the fatigue is terrible."

I left the car and joined Abby while we waited for Jolie. After the class ended, I allowed my mother to talk me through the entire ride home.

Now that I could no longer drive on highways, Jeff drove me to the city and joined my gynecological consultation. I was relieved to have company during this appointment. It became difficult to chronologically keep track of all my symptoms, especially when I focused on the most recent ones since they appeared so abruptly. My eyes burned, I experienced frequent headaches and developed a handful of colds. As a result, I missed a lot of work. I assumed these infections had more to do with a weakened immune system than having picked up something new at the pre-school. While we waited to see the doctor, Jeff held my paperwork as I napped. Anytime I sat still for more than a few minutes, my eyes closed. He tapped my shoulder when they called my name. "Trace, it's our turn."

We walked to the office, sat down and waited for the gynecologist to enter. I looked around and noticed a scattering of family pictures. I assumed the doctor was in her late forties and had two children, a son and daughter possibly in middle school.

She walked into the office, full of personality in her white coat. She was pretty, had freckles and dirty blonde curly hair. She got right to business and reviewed my chart, while asking relevant questions and listening to every story Jeff and I shared. She asked to see the results of my brain scan that was taken six months ago, but it seemed the radiologist's report wasn't sufficient. Fortunately, I had brought a copy on disc. After some time reviewing it on her computer, she turned back and asked, "Would you mind if I hold onto this? I would like to send it over to my radiologist here in the city and get a second opinion."

I nodded, "Sure."

She stood up and added, "Jeff, I hope you don't mind waiting while I take your wife to get examined." He pointed to the Golf Digest magazine he brought and insinuated he'd be fine.

During the three hour consultation—the longest we had so far—we reviewed all of the doctors' medical assessments regarding my hormones. I was impressed by her thoroughness. She asked to speak with Chris and Dr. Zacharias regarding my case and planned on sending my MRI to be reviewed.

"Clearly something is very wrong. I can tell by looking at your yellow tinted eyes, besides the distended belly."

That was the first time anyone discussed the color of my eyes. I didn't even realize they were discolored.

"I can't promise that I'll be able to solve your case but I will do my best to get you answers. I'll be in touch over the next few days with a plan."

I had a good feeling about her.

The gynecologist called two days later, confirming that I didn't have Multiple Sclerosis.

Panic ripped through my body as I sat frozen against the den couch, holding the telephone to my ear. My heart pounded all the way into my fingertips and my breath was short. This was the first doctor who had considered my diagnosis to be something permanent.

"Wait, Multiple Sclerosis? That was even a possibility?" I asked, incredulous.

She explained how some MRIs show a lesion on the brain but have nothing to do with MS. She wanted to rule it out.

I sighed in relief. Thank God I wasn't aware of that concern.

She discussed her conversations with Chris and Dr. Zacharias. Satisfied with their protocols, she focused on my hormones and the immune system.

"We want to make sure these common cold infections don't get worse and turn into something else. Rest as much as possible." She insisted I contact her if anything changed, even during the weekends.

The next morning I took Buddy back to Riker Hill Park. I awoke with a nasty cough on top of the lingering cold, but knew if I should be resting all day, Buddy needed to exercise first. While Buddy played with the other dogs, I updated Dana on my health. My neighbor overheard our conversation and asked, "Have you seen an infectious disease doctor yet?"

I laughed. "Actually that's the one category I haven't covered." She was brief with her story about someone's undiagnosed Lyme disease. They had similar symptoms and she insisted I see the same doctor. "He's a doctor with a great track record."

I watched Buddy run after a ball and leap into the air. Just as he caught it in his mouth, something struck me. Chris had mentioned something about the possibility of me having an auto-immune disorder and I stood paralyzed, wondering if it was too late to reverse my condition.

Later that night, I rested on the couch while the girls played in the basement. From a distance, I heard them laughing, and I wished I knew what made them smile. I stared in Jeff's direction with my head propped up against the pillows, and finally mustered the courage to tell him about the latest conversation at the park, hoping he would agree to another hefty expense.

"You haven't even given the gynecologist a chance! Let's see what she comes up with first," he said, after I reminded him of my MS scare.

"You don't understand. It takes forever to get consultations with these doctors and she only specializes in hormones," I stopped to catch my breath between coughs.

He looked concerned. "Are you ok?"

I took a sip of water, while trying to keep the tips of my fingers from shaking. "I'm telling you I'm getting worse. Now it's my immune system. I really think an infectious disease doctor is the way to go. I know all these doctors are so expensive but I feel like I am slowly dying here." It hurt just to blink.

He sat quietly, covering his mouth with his palm, worrying I was right. Waiting in silence, we both just stared at each other. He lowered his hand to the seat of the couch, playing with the clumps of Buddy's fur. A moment later, he looked up with a concerned look. "Have you told either doctor what you are like now?"

I nodded. "I woke up with a cough and it's gotten progressively worse." I placed my hand on my chest to stop myself from coughing. When I caught my breath, I continued, "I called both. She's going on vacation for a week but I should contact her service in an emergency," I grabbed more water to avoid another attack and shared my internist's opinion. "He wants me to call tomorrow morning if my breathing gets worse and go in for a check up."

Jeff shook his head. "Then I guess make an appointment with that doctor. You know your body best." He leaned back on the couch and massaged his forehead, taking deep breaths.

"The money is going out faster than it's coming in these days."

No truer words had been spoken between us since the mystery in my body had begun to dissolve our marriage. In fact, money was the only thing we acknowledged head on. Jeff was burdened for months now with two jobs: struggling at his own company and being Mr. Mom around the house. There was not much more I could ask from him so I closed my eyes, allowing myself to doze off before we could continue the conversation.

The cough kept me up most of the night. Two hours before school started, I found a substitute teacher to cover my shift at the pre-school. My co-workers were used to these early morning phone calls, alerting them of my absences. I probably should have taken a leave of absence but that was another form of surrender I refused to acknowledge. They felt terrible but hoped my nightmare ended soon. I resumed my position on the couch once my girls left for school. Buddy followed suit.

By ten o'clock, I found it hard to breathe. I turned off the television and focused on my symptoms. I felt heaviness around my chest. I took short and simple breaths, matching the sounds of someone on life support. This frightened me so much I called my internist. He requested that I come see him at lunch. My friend Wendy insisted she drive me to the appointment even with one of her children home sick. At first, I was stubborn and tried to refuse her offer, but she knew I was in no shape to drive.

"Don't be ridiculous. I'll be in your driveway in a half hour."

The doctor examined me right away. "Your lungs are clear but that can change very quickly." He seemed more cautious than ever as he reviewed past test results. "Call me if your breathing gets worse or anything else changes. Otherwise, rest is the best thing for you." Rest? I'd been resting for months and it seemed I still had progressively gotten worse.

I mentioned the idea of consulting an infectious disease doctor. I asked if he knew the man who came highly recommended. He had and thought it was a good idea to get another perspective, especially since my immune system had trouble fighting off respiratory infections.

I went home and made arrangements for the girls to play at their friends until Jeff got home. I didn't want them to see me in this bad of shape, and I worried my cold and cough were contagious. The last call I made for the day was to the infectious disease doctor's office. I took the first available appointment—in two weeks. I slept the rest of the day until Jeff brought the girls home.

Another bad night of sleep caused my body more fatigue. I tried to nap between my coughing attacks but was too uncomfortable. By late afternoon, I was alone and scared because of my condition. I complained to Jeff and my mother over the phone, begging for a new suggestion. They urged me to call my internist. "He's expecting you to call if you're worse."

Dr. Zacharias insisted I go to the emergency room. "I'll call the hospital, order an x-ray and blood work. I'll be in touch," he said.

Knowing I wasn't in any condition to drive myself to the hospital, I called my sister. I waited for my name to be announced and hoped Jeff showed up soon. I sat alone in the crowded waiting area. I leaned my head against the wall and looked around at the room full of strangers, praying this would be my last visit.

Two hours later, while we were waiting, Dr. Zacharias walked into my cubicle, went to the side of the bed across from Jeff, and leaned his arms against the bars. He was silent for a moment, gathering his thoughts. "So what are we going to do with you, Berko?" he asked.

I half smiled.

He shared my results. "Your lungs are clear. No pneumonia. Your lymphocytes are low but that doesn't surprise me, you've been sick. Nothing else seems abnormal." He insisted I stay in bed for the next few days to fight the infection. Gone was the jovial tone in his voice and it terrified me to hear him so serious. We shared an awkward silence.

"You're getting used to it anyway, right?" he asked, finally teasing me.

"That's for sure," I said, knowing I'd sleep most of the time. His teasing comforted me, but I wondered why this tactic no longer worked for my husband.

My coworker's oldest daughter was having a Bat Mitzvah that same weekend. This was a good friend who was about to celebrate a major milestone with her family and I couldn't be a part of it. I had no doubt that everyone understood my situation, never thinking twice about my disappearances. Though I was tired of missing important social events and disappointing my friends and family, I listened to the doctor's orders and stayed in bed through the weekend, which gave me a lot of time to think. As I lay there hour after hour, I realized how frustrated I was waiting for some-one to give me a diagnosis, and I decided it was time to take matters into my own hands.

When I wasn't sleeping, I researched all possibilities for a diagnosis on my computer. I used every combination of symptoms in search words. I hoped to find the website that would change my life and cure me. Who needed a doctor when I had scientific information at my disposal? It made no difference if I typed in one, two or three symptoms at a time. The results proved the same. When I keyed in any hormonal symptoms, I was led to websites for women experiencing hypothyroidism or menopause, both dead ends.

I shifted directions and checked out illnesses I had heard the doctors briefly mention: Lyme Disease, Lupus and other auto-immune deficiencies. It was hard to decipher between them when

I had at least three of the symptoms for each illness. I refocused my efforts around the worst symptoms: chronic fatigue, weight gain and respiratory infections, and found a book by James Wilson called *Adrenal Fatigue: The 21st Century Stress Syndrome*. I had every symptom. I hollered from the bedroom for Jeff to come hear my discovery.

"You'll never believe this but I think I found my diagnosis."

He barely stood in the doorway, looking doubtful. Yet, he listened.

Over the next ten minutes, I read him numerous paragraphs until he lost interest.

"Sounds like what you've been experiencing but I never heard of that." He was brief and eager to go back to the den where Buddy rested.

It was another long weekend for Jeff. For nine months, he had cared for the girls and Buddy without much help on my part. When Jeff was home, he spent most of his time in the den, the opposite side of the house from me, and his visits to our bedroom had become less frequent. When he did appear, he stood at the foot of the bed, occasionally placing his hand on the top of the duvet cover by my feet. The second I looked away, his hand was gone, leaving me with a deeper sense of guilt. I had done little to make the situation easier on him and it was evident that our intimacy was deteriorating with the distance I put between us. It had been a year since we brought Buddy home. A year since we had really felt like a couple.

"You should mention all this to the gynecologist the next time you speak with her," he said, closing the door behind him.

I was going to do more than mention it. Somehow, I was going to prove it.

I headed to Barnes and Noble that Monday morning with all ten pages printed from the website and with the help of the sales clerk, found James Wilson's book on Adrenal Fatigue. I grabbed as many other books I could find on the same topic. My legs felt weak so I sat down on the floor, opened my notebook and took copious notes, searching and searching until something struck me. I could hardly believe my eyes. Right there in black and white was the answer to my prayers. *Steroids were used as a cure!* I bought Wilson's book, left and called my mother.

"Oh my god, mom. I think I found my diagnosis! I can't believe it. I'm freaking out and there's a way to get better."

I rambled on about Adrenal Fatigue, its symptoms and the benefit of steroids.

"I don't care if I never heard of it," my mother cried, elated to hear my spirits lifted. "I can't wait to tell your father. We'll get you those steroids. Don't you worry!"

I couldn't wait to share this news with the medical team.

CHAPTER
15

B Y THE TIME I went to my next acupuncture treatment on Thursday, I was prepared to pitch my latest discovery. Chris walked in holding my thick file of paperwork. I held up the cover to James Wilson's book and rambled on about Adrenal Fatigue. Chris confirmed my suspicions, explaining why he had been supporting my adrenal glands with supplements, hoping to give them a chance to rest and get back into balance. Over the last six months, he had mentioned the imbalance of my adrenal glands, but I never connected the dots to Adrenal Fatigue until then.

"I've read that steroids revive the adrenals. I want to try that," I said.

As a holistic practitioner, Chris was less than enthusiastic over the use of steroids, since it was another form of a hormone with negative side effects. I changed topics, and complained of my new symptoms: joint pain in my hands, legs and feet, coupled with tender points on my body when pressure was applied. It appeared this was the onset of fibromyalgia, which is a complicated condition of combined muscle fatigue and inflammation. In short, it is the body's inability to recover from daily stressors. He suggested I take two new supplements, hoping they would relieve some discomfort, and administered another acupuncture treatment. I slept most of the session, feeling like I had just won the jackpot. In no time at all, I'd be cured and have my life back.

My elation continued through the week. A rush of euphoria guided me and I needed to use every bit of that energy to win back my girls. Ever since our trip to New York City, I'd catch them looking at me with skepticism, and it bothered me that they thought I might be like 'this' forever. When my girls came home from school later that week, they were excited to find workmen assembling their new trampoline in the backyard. I didn't care that their present was delivered a month before their birthday. I wanted to be a hero, even for a day.

After dinner, I rested on the deck furniture and watched the girls jump for more than an hour. Buddy ran in circles with feral energy while the girls giggled and played games on the trampoline. I had totally given up training him by the end of June and, like me, he had sensed his new freedom—though his would far outlast mine. Jolie teased and gently pushed her face against the trampoline net. "Look at me, Boo. I bet you can't jump this high." He stopped and seemed interested, then got distracted by the squirrel running underneath and chased after it.

Abby hollered, "Mom, can you jump with us? It's so much fun."

"I don't feel up to jumping, sweetie." I wish I did. I hated using my sickness as an excuse, but it was the only explanation I could give. I wish it had been an excuse for something. It was a constant, nagging state of being that left me with little patience and plagued me with guilt. "Besides you only have five more minutes before you have to shower," I said, seeing the girls' disappointment. I assumed my 'hero for a day' role had ended.

When the girls finished playing outside, they showered, got into pajamas and sat on their beds as Jeff read books. I lay in bed and listened to my family through the master bedroom wall, saddened that Jeff had replaced me again in another one of my favorite maternal duties. I was bummed when I heard Jolie shout, "Dad, let's pick an age. Tell us a story from when you were eight." That was my game I created with the girls. They'd pick an age and I told them a story from childhood before I tucked them into bed. I gave the usual hugs and kisses, turned their light off and finished with a phrase from an old movie. "I love you always, always, forever, forever." Now they gave the kisses, tucked me into bed, and closed my bedroom door behind them.

I spent another weekend napping on and off, while Jeff, the girls and Buddy enjoyed the trampoline in the backyard. I regretted choosing the location outside our bedroom window. No matter how hard I tried to sleep, there was no way I could avoid hearing them play. The girls were having a blast as Jeff bounced them high in the air. Between the laughter, shrieks, and Buddy's barking, I woke up.

On the way to the bathroom, I stopped and leaned against our half-opened window to watch my family, wondering if they missed me. I longed for enjoyment and connection, lamenting that the few moments I had with them over the last year were not enough to sustain me. A little over a year, Buddy passed his puppy stage and his body had gotten stronger and bigger. This would have been the opportune time for Buddy to handle long distance runs. Instead,

I watched him roam the backyard, forgetting the commands I had spent hours teaching him the prior summer. It seemed as if I was disappearing even faster from my family's mind and I worried if my health continued to decline, I'd be left alone for good.

A week later, I saw the gynecologist and pitched her my potential diagnosis of Adrenal Fatigue. She agreed without hesitation, but needed proof and ordered a thorough metabolic blood panel. I hoped the results exposed my low levels of cortisol, indicating Adrenal Fatigue, and I wondered if my cortisol levels would be more precise with a saliva test versus a blood test. She planned to test the complete metabolic breakdown of my body, which would take a week.

"If you have adrenal fatigue, this should cover it," she said, refusing to recommend steroids yet.

While I was convinced I had Adrenal Fatigue, I was eager to hear from the infectious disease doctor. I booked a late morning consultation and Jeff agreed to meet me before the appointment in front of the hospital where the doctor's office was located. Earlier that morning, I organized my health records and made sure all eighty pages were present; however, I left the folder on the counter with my car keys and handbag.

Just before I left the house, Buddy scratched at the sliding doors in the kitchen. I hollered, "Really, you have to go hurry ups now?" Done with his accidents, I placed my bag and paperwork down, and sent him outside. "Be quick, Bud. I can't be late."

When I reopened the sliding door, Buddy galloped to get inside and trotted ahead of me, wanting to play. I was in too much of a hurry to engage him and tripped over him when I turned to grab my things from the counter.

"Watch out, Boo!" I said, rolling my eyes for the umpteenth time in his presence.

He backed up an inch and sat down, staring at me, sensing my frustration. I couldn't resist his droopy eyes and rubbed his head, feeling ashamed of neglecting him.

I sighed, "I'm sorry, Boo." He lifted his paw and placed it on my hand, knocking my car key to the floor. As I bent down, I felt a shooting pain in my kneecaps and hips, reminding me why I needed help. At this point, Buddy took whatever attention I gave him, even if it was only for a minute. I reached for my bag and gated Buddy into the kitchen before leaving the house.

When I parked at the hospital, I realized the folder was missing from the passenger seat. I looked on the floor and quickly turned, hoping it was on the back seat—but I had clearly left it behind at the house. With less than a half hour before my consultation, I had nothing to show the new doctor. I leaned back against the driver's seat, shaking my head. I was losing my mind. Not only was my body unrecognizable, my brain wasn't functioning the way it used to—another indication that something was very wrong. I had never thought my mental ability was being affected by my condition until now. Though I had read nothing that would indicate this was true, I wondered if a disturbed endocrine system could negatively affect my mind.

In tears, I called Jeff and rambled hysterically. Frustrated by my forgetfulness, he stopped at the house, grabbed the folder and met me at the doctor's office.

We were finally seated in a small cramped room with a balding doctor, trying to hear him above the window air conditioner for twenty minutes. He looked up from my file and said, "You definitely have something, but I can't put my finger on it."

I looked at Jeff, exchanging a knowing look as if to say, here we go again. Someone, please cue the music.

"I think the Mayo Clinic is the way to go," he said and gave the phone number for the gastroenterology department at the Minnesota clinic and told me to follow-up with him in six weeks. I balked at the thought of returning to his office.

Jeff and I walked to the elevator in silence. Once we got inside Jeff said, "We spent more time in his waiting room than with him." He sighed while hitting the button for the lobby. "How much did that just cost us?"

This time I was just as frustrated. "Three-hundred sixty dollars to hear him say I have something but he can't put his finger on it," I shook my head in disbelief. "Now what?"

The elevator doors opened and we stepped out into the hall in order to take a different elevator to the garage.

"You're definitely not giving him any more of our money for a twenty minute appointment!"

I stared at him, vexed, while the next elevator doors closed behind us. Did he not have enough faith in my own decision-making and believe I'd run back to this doctor any time soon?

"You think the Mayo Clinic is going to be less expensive?" I asked, feeling my stomach sink when the elevator descended into the bowels of the parking garage.

He didn't respond. We walked to my car in silence and Jeff kissed my forehead as I got into my car. "Go home and rest. I love you."

I shut the car door and turned on the ignition, fighting tears. This did not feel like love.

I got on the highway and dialed my mother. When my dad answered their house phone, I knew he was eager for a chance to catch up with me. Before my sickness, I'd be just as enthusiastic to hear his voice. My relationship with him was as open and honest as my mother's, sharing mostly the same information minus the girly stuff. Now things were different and all he had to hear was my tone of voice before asking, "Are you looking for Mom?"

I assumed he'd be disappointed to miss any opportunity to speak with his daughter. My intentions weren't to dash his hopes but I had a one-track mind when consumed with sadness and needed to hear my mother's voice. It didn't matter how many times we spoke, she'd always answer me with optimism and skillfully handle my tantrums as they arose. I reiterated the doctor's visit, sharing my concerns about the Mayo Clinic. "If I go there, I could be gone for up to two weeks. Who would take care of the girls and how much is that stay going to cost?"

Regardless of the money, she insisted I call and try to get accepted. She had the foresight to see beyond my obstacles. I continued, "We haven't even been reimbursed for any of the out-of-network consultations because we have yet to hit our deductible. What's the point of paying an insurance premium every year if these doctors don't take insurance? Not to mention how much money we spent on all those supplements."

She interrupted, "If we have to, Dad and I will help pay for the doctor bills. You need to get well. That's the priority." Although I felt guilty, I thanked her for being supportive. She finished, "Hang up and call the Mayo Clinic now and let me know what happens."

After some debate, I listened and spent ten minutes on hold before being transferred to the gastroenterology department. Finally, I got a live voice on the phone an spoke to a secretary. I pitched a five-minute health recap, including all my symptoms and emphasizing the severity of my bloat and constipation. She thought my symptoms didn't match their department's guidelines and suggested I try the endocrinology department, since I was taking thyroid medication and had gained excessive weight—thirty pounds to be exact.

When she transferred me, I lost cell service and got disconnected while holding for the new department. I dialed again and waited another ten minutes to speak with someone, feeling the heat of short-tempered sparks flaring. Lately, even the littlest things such as a dropped phone call irritated me and I blamed my actions on the fatigue.

I was relieved to hear a live voice. I tweaked my pitch, emphasizing symptoms that fell under their department. With thyroid issues, weak adrenal glands, the change in metabolism and hormonal issues, I expected to get approval. Apparently, it wasn't as easy as I imagined.

The secretary requested I fax my records for the doctors to review. If I faxed everything today, I would hear from their office within two to three days. If I mailed my records, it would be a two-week turnaround before I received word. The last thing I felt like doing was another errand. Two hours out of the house each day was enough for my body, but the idea of waiting any longer for a diagnosis was more than I could bear.

I hung up and drove directly to Staples. I leaned against the fax machine for support, feeding it eighty pages, one page at a time, after the first attempt jammed the machine. At this point, my frustration peaked and I was seconds from a full-blown meltdown, recalling the times when my daughters, as toddlers, had missed their morning naps and burst into tantrums. I longed for my bed. The only thing that kept me composed was knowing that my girls would be starting camp the following week, and I'd have nine hours each day to sleep on the couch without any guilt. It was a good thing Buddy couldn't speak.

The next afternoon, I overheard Jeff speaking with one of his golf buddies, declining another golf game. He hadn't asked me to play in the longest time. I was anxious to hear his explanation. I leaned against the wall while he spoke, trying to stay hidden. There was no disguising the bleakness in his voice and the desperation to join his friends on the course.

Since Jeff was twelve, he played golf and made the college team his freshman year of school. After he graduated and moved to New York, he joined a country club within a half hour from his apartment, spending most weekends on the golf course with his friends. He was great at it and loved the game. It was his form of exercise and a way to unwind. I knew it was a huge part of his life, just as running became mine and we allotted time each weekend to accommodate both of our needs. That freedom dwindled as my health declined, leaving him without a way to release unneeded stress. Hearing his disappointment, my chest felt tight with guilt, knowing I was the sole reason he had no free time to play with his friends and release any stress.

Like most men in his situation, he coped with his powerlessness by compartmentalizing it to stay afloat and keep us going. He followed my lead most days and stayed quiet while he witnessed his spouse suffer. Both of us wanted to fix the whole situation, but we had no control over any of it. Without a network of girlfriends and consistent lunches like me, Jeff's support system consisted of his buddies on the golf course, who he'd seen once in the last few months.

After he hung up the phone, I sat down at the kitchen table. I stared at him while he made the girls lunch. Silence filled the room. My spurts of anger, fear and resentment had taken a toll on Jeff and left him quiet in my presence most times. He deserved some space and a chance away from this madness. I felt like I owed him that much. I heard him say the tee time was for early Sunday morning and since camp started the following day, I could rest more then.

"I think you should play golf with the guys tomorrow morning," I said, offering this small gesture of love, maybe the first I had been able to give him in months.

Jeff swung around to face me, his facial expression all lit up. "Really? Are you sure you'd be okay with that?" he asked. His eyes widened, and he smiled, full of hope.

I nodded. "It's only a few hours. Just take Buddy for a walk when you get back."

"Okay!" It was nice to see him excited about something for once. He grabbed the girls' plates of tuna fish and looked back at me. "You're sure you're feeling up to it?"

I appreciated his thoughtfulness. "It's fine, really, I want you to have some fun," I said, realizing the girls would be sleeping for a few hours while he was gone. I could handle five hours on my own.

After Jeff left for golf that Sunday morning, Abby woke up not feeling well. Her eyes looked glassy, her skin pale, and she was extremely weak with a fever of 102 degrees. This isn't happening, I thought. Not on the only day that Jeff could golf. Murphy's Law was dictating our lives—in an absurdly comic way. Since Abby wouldn't eat any breakfast, I gave her an orange flavored Gatorade to keep her hydrated. While she watched television, I napped next to her on the couch. Jolie played with her American Girl dolls on the carpet and chased Buddy, who snagged their Webkins every chance he got.

Abby whined, "Mommy, wake up." I blinked, trying to open my eyes, unsure how long I had drifted off. I was inches from Abby, hearing her voice but could not answer her no matter how hard I tried. No words came out of my mouth and I panicked when I heard her cry.

"Mom, please, I don't feel good. Wake up."

I was desperate to lift my body but it was dead weight. I couldn't move. Abby began to cough. Then a loud burp turned into a gagging sound. Oh God, I thought, knowing what was coming next.

I fought to open my eyes. Everything was blurry, but once it cleared, I saw her sitting upright, leaning over the edge of the couch, tears falling down her cheeks and orange saliva dripping from her mouth. I looked down at the carpet, seeing her pile of vomit.

I sighed, "Oh, Ab. You really don't feel good, huh?"

She whimpered, "I'm sorry I got it on the carpet but I tried to wake you."

"I know, honey. I heard you but I just couldn't move."

We stared at each other, incredulous at this mother-daughter quagmire. It was one thing not to be able to help myself, but to see my own child struggling was the worst consequence of my condition. I wanted to reach out and hold her, do something to comfort her, but all I could do was stare. I hated that I had not only become sick but utterly useless in her eyes.

She dry heaved some more, then mumbled, "I think I'm going to be sick again." Abby was ten feet from our den bathroom and knew I was in no shape to help. She looked at me, shook her head and said, "I can't make it." I glanced over at Jolie who was staring back at me. Her little face filled with worry. Jolie's biggest fear was getting the stomach virus. She hated to vomit. It was clear she'd stay as far away from Abby as possible. It would be hours before Jeff returned. I needed him immediately and was pissed that I let him leave.

I closed my eyes and took a deep breath, then mustered every ounce of strength I had left to push myself off the couch, stand and carry Abby to the toilet. Ten feet felt like a mile, but I refused to give up, grateful that whatever was inside me had not stolen my resolve to be a mother who cared. It might have made me overweight, fatigued and irritable, but I would be damned before it made me apathetic.

I sat down on the floor next to Abby, leaning against the wall and held her hair back while she was sick. I realized this could be more than just a stomach virus. There were different strains of the flu going around and many of my friends' kids had it. When we were both able to leave the bathroom, I immediately called our pediatrician. He insisted I bring her in right away to start her on Tamiflu. I called Jeff's cell but got his voicemail and decided I would drive the girls myself, even in my exhausted state—this time with the windows open and music blasting.

When we arrived in the parking lot, Abby couldn't move. The tips of her brown hair were wet from sweating and stuck to her face. She cried, "Please, carry me. I can't walk."

I took a deep breath, bit my tongue and picked her up, knowing it was hard enough to walk around with the extra thirty-five pounds currently from my sickness. Jolie was silent, walking on the opposite side of my hip that held Abby. I wasn't even halfway to the pediatrician's office before tears dripped down my face. I wasn't sure how much more I could handle, silently resenting Jeff's absence.

We returned home an hour later with a bottle of Tamiflu. The moment Jeff got home, I left the den and got into bed immediately, terrified of my deteriorating immune system and the uncalled-for attitude toward him. I slept most of the afternoon. With Abby home sick that first week of camp, my nine hours of guilt-free sleep were gone. The only upside? Someone else was around to pay attention to Buddy.

CHAPTER
16

D URING THE LAST WEEK IN JUNE, the gynecologist called with my results. I stared out my kitchen window as she explained, "While some of your levels are low, they're not low enough to prove Adrenal Fatigue." I closed my eyes, realizing I hit another roadblock.

I begged, "Would you still consider prescribing steroids? I can't live like this anymore. It's been over a year since I've been sick and I'm only getting worse. Can I at least give it a try?"

She was silent for a moment, wavering after she heard the despair in my voice. She offered to speak with my internist to make a joint decision. I hoped they connected before July 4th weekend. I didn't want to cancel more plans.

Later that week, my internist called with the good news. "I spoke to your gynecologist and we're starting you on five milligrams of Cortef."

I was elated. "Oh my god, really?" I shut my eyes for a quick minute. Was that light I saw finally burning away the darkness? I wanted to reach out and hug this doctor.

"It's a low dose and we'll have to increase it next week, but let's see how you feel then. I sent the prescription to your pharmacy."

One hour later, I took my first pill and believed I'd be back to my old self in no time.

July 4th weekend, I woke up early Saturday and glanced over at the clock. It was 7:30. The house was silent other than the rhythmic sound of Jeff snoring. This was the first time in months I woke before my family, feeling well-rested.

As I looked around the bedroom, something felt different. My eyes didn't burn anymore. I blinked an extra few times just to relish this small feat. Immediately, I checked my hands. I clenched them to make a fist. Then I spread my fingers. The throbbing sensations were gone. I was baffled by this change and continued to check the rest of my body. My ankles turned easily and effortlessly. I could also lift my legs without pain. I took a deep breath, feeling my smile widen. I slid my hands over my abdomen, praying it, too, would be healed. My basketball-sized belly was still very real but it wasn't stopping me from going on a run. This was going to be one fantastic Independence Day weekend.

I hopped out of bed to wash my face and brush my teeth. Normal hygiene tasks had gotten difficult for me, but that was over now. I brushed my teeth with the finesse of a seasoned dental hygienist. I smiled at myself. Things were looking up. After all this time, I was about to hit the pavement—called life—and put this all behind me. I threw on tight gym clothes, figuring a month of my old exercise regimen combined with my new food plan would help me lose the weight in no time. I tied the last lace to my sneakers, grabbed my iPod and left the house.

There wasn't a cloud in the sky. It was hot and sticky outside but nothing stopped my determination to get reacquainted with the pavement. I listened to one of my favorite songs, "Brand New Day" by Joshua Radin. I blasted the volume and ran, focusing on the beauty of the outdoors: the green lawns, flowers in bloom and my moving legs. This was *my* brand new day.

It wasn't long before I lost stamina, after hearing three songs from my playlist. I used to handle a four-mile run with ease, but now ten minutes was hard enough to complete. Since this was my first attempt, I took it easy and walked back to the house, excited to share my news.

When I returned, everyone was still asleep. I raced to my bedroom and jumped on top of Jeff and shouted, "Guess what I just did?" He needed a second to open his eyes and squinted, staring back at me. I was inches away from his face, probably the closest we had been in months. I continued, "I ran—outdoors. And ok, so I could only do it for ten minutes but it felt incredible to move again. It's a miracle, it's like I woke up from a coma!"

Jeff was in shock and needed a minute to process this change. It had been a year since he'd seen me with this much energy. He glanced at my arms, which were holding the rest of my body above him, aware of the change in my strength.

"You think it's the steroid? You've only been on it a few days." He wiped the corners of his eyes from sleepiness.

I got off the bed in quick strides. In a cheerful tone I said, "Absolutely. I told you I had Adrenal Fatigue and I just needed the steroid to get better. And now I'm better." I couldn't stop moving and found myself pacing on his side of the bed.

"That's great, hon." He fluffed his pillows and sat up, grabbing the remote and turned on the television.

I headed towards the door. "Wait until I tell the girls." I didn't look back and shouted, "I'll feed everyone breakfast, including Buddy. It's been too long."

The girls were happy to see I was full of energy and thrilled to be waited on hand and foot. I appreciated the ability to sit upright at the kitchen table without any effort. After breakfast, they got dressed. Abby walked into the kitchen while I was doing the dishes.

"Now that you're feeling better, would you go on the trampoline with us?"

I hesitated and placed the last glass into the dishwasher. I turned around and saw the hope on her sweet face. She was dressed in a tanktop and frayed cut off jean shorts. Her thick hair was combed neatly and pulled into a high ponytail. She was ready to play.

"Last one to the trampoline is a rotten egg," I said and winked.

Her face beamed as she jumped up and down. I grabbed a paper towel, wiped my hands and opened the sliding doors. Buddy darted for the door, pushing my leg aside.

Abby shouted towards the bedrooms, "Oh my god, Jolie, mom's going on the trampoline with us!"

Jolie ran into the kitchen, dressed in a different outfit than Abby's, her hair pushed back by a headband. "No, she's not." She looked at me then glanced over at Abby and back at me. She continued, "Are you serious?" Her face lit up as she watched Buddy and me head towards the trampoline.

She skipped her way onto the grass. "Wait for me!"

At first, I ran in circles with Buddy, playing his favorite game of chase. I stopped rather quickly because I was out of breath, then grabbed a tennis ball and tossed it in the air. "Fetch, Boo," I said, watching Buddy gallop across the lawn. The ball landed before he caught it, which left him roaming the area.

"It's behind you," I said, chuckling, hoping that *all of this* was finally behind us. I was no longer sick in that moment and I felt as though my whole life had returned instantaneously.

When Buddy finally found the ball, he picked it up with his mouth and trotted back, stopping ten feet away from me. He rested on all fours, dropping the ball between his front two paws while his tail swished side to side, awaiting my next move. I commanded, "Buddy, come!" He did not budge. I repeated the command and watched as his body stayed motionless.

"Come on Mom," Jolie said, pressing her face against the trampoline net. After my third command and no response, I laughed and joined the girls. It was another reminder that I was no longer his master. But I didn't care. I finally had enough energy to play with him and my family.

The girls took turns jumping solo while I sat on the edge of the trampoline. A few minutes later, it was my turn. They sat towards the middle, hoping I bounced them high into the air like the game they played with Jeff, one I had only seen from a distance since we had gotten them the trampoline. Jolie insisted, "Now let's all jump at the same time holding hands."

The first few jumps were soft and slow, trying to get in sync with each other. The higher we jumped, the harder it was for the girls to stay balanced. It was inevitable that one of them would fall. Their grins and laughter warmed my heart. God, I missed these special moments. I got choked up and teary-eyed, realizing I wasn't watching from my bedroom window any longer or fearing a future without them.

I let go of their hands and wiped my eyes. Abby asked, "Mom, are you crying?"

"What? No," I said and turned away to cover my face. "Something just flew into one of my eyes." I had gotten used to hiding my emotions over the past year, though I'm not sure everything went undetected. My girls were smart and I could feel their eyes on me.

Jeff stuck his head out the screen door and asked if everyone wanted to swim at the club. Though I was relieved to have their attention on something else, I wasn't too excited to squeeze my body into a bathing suit that barely fit, but went inside to change while Jeff walked Buddy.

I pulled out two new one-piece bathing suits from my dresser, wishing I'd still fit into my old two-piece suits instead. I tried on both and looked in the mirror, examining the excess weight. A dreadful sensation filled my body. Suddenly, I didn't know who I was seeing in the mirror. Everything about how I felt on the inside at that moment did not match what I saw on the outside. I wanted to look as fabulous as I felt. The steroids weren't working fast enough.

Disappointed, I ripped off the second suit, changed clothes, hopped into bed and turned on the television. Here I was thrilled to feel alive again but was sucked back into a black hole.

A few minutes later, Jeff found me in bed. "What are you doing? I thought you were getting dressed?" I shared my frustrations and hoped he'd go without me.

He took a deep breath.

"Who cares what you look like. Just throw on one of those bathing suits and you'll relax on a lounge chair."

I lifted my eyes and stared at him. After all the times he's seen me tormented over my body size, that was all he could say to comfort me? Apparently, the answer was yes.

I whined. "I can't take it. I don't recognize myself anymore."

"You got to get past the weight gain and give the steroids a chance to work. It's been a long time since you've been this energized. We're spending the day as a family."

He was right. I got dressed, changed my attitude and looked forward to the afternoon. Even if I would have to wear a suit four sizes bigger than me, I was going to enjoy my family.

🐾 🐾

It was the first full day of weekend plans I had in months. Between my short run, time spent at the pool and hours out of bed, I was tired. The steroid only helped so much. By Saturday night of July 4th, Jeff and I drove home from dinner in silence. I stared out the window, praying for more strength and assumed he kept quiet, hoping to avoid an argument.

We walked into the house and I made small talk with the babysitter, catching up on the night's activities, the games played, conversations shared and actual bedtime, knowing they usually convinced their sitters to stay up longer. I didn't care all that much. I wanted them to have fun. Then I asked for the update on Buddy. In the babysitter's eyes, he could do no wrong. She loved dogs and gave him plenty of attention.

"I forgot to tell you what Buddy did tonight. It was so crazy," she said on her way out.

I felt a pit in my stomach and immediately looked down at her feet. The last sitter left our house missing half of her flip-flop. He ate a chunk of it while she played with the girls in the basement. Hesitant, I asked, "Uh oh, what did he do?"

She giggled. "I sat in the den, watching television from the middle of the couch. Buddy grabbed your chenille blanket off the floor with his teeth and dragged it over to me, covering my whole lap. It was pretty cool. Has he ever done that to you guys?"

I quickly responded, "No." Even the babysitter gave him more attention. Now I was really far down on his list of favorites. As she repeated the story to Jeff, it hit me. "That's the exact position I sat in every day since I've been sick, with a blanket wrapped around my legs!"

Amazed, I turned to Jeff and asked, "Can a dog notice that?" We were all shocked.

"I've never seen a dog do that before but obviously, he noticed," the babysitter said. I smiled and nodded awkwardly. Most days I forgot Buddy was even in the same room.

The positive effects of steroids were short lived. Over the next two weeks, my internist increased the dosage two different times, but nothing relieved my symptoms. My joints ached, my eyes burned and the exhaustion slowly crept back. The higher the dose, the more weight I gained.

One morning, I got dressed in gym clothes and headed outside for a run. It had been so long since I felt the positive effects of a workout. As I left the bedroom, Jeff insisted I stop exercising altogether.

"I know in your heart you want to run but your body says otherwise."

I stared at him a moment, thinking *oh no, mister. You might control the finances in this situation, but I'm controlling how and when I decide to use my body for something that I can actually enjoy.* I refused to let my chronic condition win and ran on willpower instead.

I turned on my iPod, blasted the music and headed down the street. Every step I took resulted in throbbing sensations throughout my legs. I ignored the pain for the first thirty steps. By the time I reached the house next door, my legs gave out. I lost all balance and fell to the ground, using my hands to break the fall. Frightened, I pulled myself onto the sidewalk and checked for bruises. My left palm had a quarter-sized raspberry while my left knee was scraped.

I looked up at the sky, broke down and cried, questioning my fate and refusing to acknowledge that Jeff had warned me to stop. *Why me?* I thought. *What did I do to deserve this?*

Tears dripped off my cheeks as I glanced down the street. I hunched over and swayed, feeling the surge of anger rising within me. I grabbed the largest pebble I could find and hurled it with whatever strength I had left, wishing to detonate the darkness.

"Am I supposed to live this way forever?" I asked, looking up at the clear blue sky.

I took a breath. Weeping, I said, "Someone, help me." I received no answers. "Please!"

I got up and slowly walked back to the house with my head hanging in defeat. I went straight into my bedroom, whimpering as I pushed open the door. Jeff was in bed, watching ESPN News. Startled, he looked at me while tears erupted again.

"What happened?" he asked and sat up.

In between short breaths, I blurted, "I fell while trying to run. I didn't even make it past the neighbor's house, I've got nothing left in me."

His brow furrowed. "Are you ok? Did you hurt yourself?"

I turned my palms away from him, not wanting to call attention to the bruises. "Do I look ok? I've gained almost forty freaking pounds, Jeff. I can't run anymore and I always feel like crap."

He sat silently, afraid to offer a suggestion, knowing he'd be attacked despite his good intentions. Jeff resented the fact that he had to walk on eggshells when I was around. Even then, his patience astounded me, but I had no way of pausing for a moment to acknowledge that. The triggers had been pushed and I was ready for a fight. If I couldn't spar with the Big Guy in the Sky, I could slug my husband with my poor attitude, right? My anger reared its ugly head.

"If this is what my future is going to be like…" I stopped mid-sentence.

"Then what?" he asked in a stern tone. His eyes pierced mine and the TV went off. I had never seen him look at me with disdain. "We're doing everything we can for you to get better! You have to stay strong. I get it's not easy but what other choice do you have?"

I lifted an arm and wiped my cheeks. "You don't get it! What if someone cut off your arm and you could never play golf again?

How would you deal?" I was shaking. "I hate my life, myself," I said, looking away and paused. "I hate us!"

I turned back slowly, afraid to see his expression.

He went pale and looked shocked, then leaned forward in the bed. "What do you mean by that? You hate us."

I met his gaze. It felt like it was all over. Just like that.

Our connection was gone. Even though we were a good team for twelve years, had each other's backs, prioritized the same values and enjoyed our time together, I could no longer deny who we had become as a couple. It was as if we spoke a different language and lived on separate continents. Every time he touched me, I cringed and moved away, assuming my change of heart was obvious to him. Of course I missed the old us—the light-hearted conversations, the passion and the desire to be wanted, but that felt like eons ago. It seemed Jeff was most concerned with our finances and lack of sex life. I was suffocating and stayed quiet too long.

"If this is what our life together will be like, then I don't want it anymore. I'm done! I just want to leave," I said, raising a hand, rubbing the bridge of my nose. I looked up again.

"I want a divorce!"

Tears filled Jeff's eyes. "Do you seriously mean that?"

I didn't. I still loved my husband. I wasn't ready for that next step: separate homes, divorce lawyers and splitting the girls time between us, but emotions had hit a wall. I sobbed, "I just feel trapped inside, like I'm in a prison and wished there was a way to escape this mess." I didn't admit that I had considered living with my parents for a while but I couldn't leave the girls.

I heard a voice from behind. "I'm hungry. Can I have breakfast?" It was Abby, standing at our bedroom door. My eyes widened and my heart sank wondering if she witnessed any part of our conversation.

Jeff flipped the covers off his legs and stood up. "I'll give you breakfast, sweetie." He walked past me and straight for the door.

I couldn't turn around and face my daughter. It seemed as if I kept letting my family down, day after day. Abby asked, "Mom, you okay?"

I shook my head, took a deep breath and answered, "Yep. I'm fine." They headed to the kitchen while I walked to the bathroom. Alone, I slowly sunk to floor, sliding against the wall and cried.

A few minutes later, Buddy appeared at the edge of the bathroom door. He got down on all fours and stared at me. I looked back while wiping my tears. He didn't blink, his big brown eyes as wide and open as his heart. I wondered what he was thinking, if he resented me, too, wishing my heart would be as open to him. There are precious moments in a lifetime that we can connect with animals, and this was one of those times when I knew Buddy had come from a special place that I might never understand. We stared at each other, but I didn't say a word.

"Hon, where are you?" Jeff asked.

In a muffled voice, I responded. "In the bathroom." He came in a moment later and smiled when he saw Buddy keeping me company.

Jeff climbed over him and sat down next to me. He placed his arm around my neck, leaning my head against his chest and turned to Buddy. "You're making 'the mommy' feel better, Boo?" Buddy moved closer and laid his head on Jeff's lap, hoping to get rubbed. Then he flipped over and rested on his back while Jeff massaged his belly.

"Would you look at this dog?"

My heart rate slowed while he rubbed Buddy's neck, grateful for the goodness in my husband's heart. "He's amazing. Talk about unconditional love," I said and reached out to stroke Buddy's face, then bent down and kissed his snout. I lifted my head and looked into Jeff's eyes. "I didn't mean what I said. I'm just scared that I'm never getting better and I'm so tired of being miserable."

Jeff took it in and nodded. "Me too."

I laughed and Jeff raised his hand, carefully touching the strands of hair that had fallen out of my ponytail and wrapped them behind my ear. He smiled when I didn't pull away.

"I don't know anyone else that could have handled this year the way you did," he said and kissed my forehead. He pulled my head against his chest and I could hear his heart pounding. "We'll get a diagnosis, Trace. Just don't give up on us. Deal?"

I nodded, happy to feel his embrace. We both desperately needed this intimacy.

Buddy turned back on his belly and stretched out his front paws. I grabbed onto one and asked, "Do you think Abby heard me?" Jeff was confident she heard nothing. I looked down at Buddy as he raised his eyebrows, imploring us for some playtime. "He could really use *a you know what,*" I said, always careful with my choice of words around him.

"I'll take him," Jeff said and kissed the top of my head again.

"Boo, you want to go for a walk?" Buddy jumped up and darted out of the room. We heard the sounds of galloping paws as he raced down the hallway. Jeff went to get his leash.

I took another minute before I got up from the bathroom floor. I looked in the mirror and washed my face, trying to rid any evidence of a meltdown. I went straight to my closet. I slowly knelt, avoiding any excess pain in my legs and reached behind a rack of clothes, scanning through the stack of shoeboxes, trying to find the one for my sneakers. I loosened the laces and pulled them out, placing each shoe inside the box, wondering if I'd ever find something as satisfying as my morning runs. I took a deep breath, closed the lid, and shoved the box in the back of the closet. I got up and headed for the hallway, seeing my first and only half-marathon plaque with my photo hanging on the wall. I stopped to touch the photo picturing me with my arms held high when I crossed the finish line. I believed those days were over and I wondered if there would ever be a finish line to cross with my condition.

A few days later, I sat in my internist's office and begged for a new direction. He rummaged through my file and rechecked the many blood test results on his computer, hoping something new appeared, but he was at a loss. I reiterated my twenty-minute consultation with the infectious disease doctor and shared my latest devastating news. "I heard from the Mayo Clinic. I don't fit under any department's criteria, so there goes that idea. Now what?"

Anytime I discussed my health, I ended in tears. He handed me the box of tissues that was on his desk and leaned back in his chair. He stared at me.

"I'm not sure."

"I really thought that steroids would cure me." I took a breath, wiped my tears and continued, "I've seen more than ten different specialists in fourteen months, been to the emergency room a handful of times and nobody has a clue. My family is falling apart. Jeff's frustrated, the girls hate me and I don't blame them. I can't live like this much longer. Just tell me what type of specialist to see and I'll find the best."

At this point, he knew my options were limited. He started from scratch and focused on the first symptoms I experienced: excessive bloating, constipation and fatigue. We sat silent. A few minutes later, he suggested, "There's a doctor in the city who's a great diagnostician. He spoke at a conference I attended. I think he may be one of the few options left. His name is Dr. Leo Galland." He Googled the doctor's name on the computer and found his website. I wrote down his name and number after learning that Dr. Galland was an award-winning pioneer in the field of Functional Medicine. I hoped this doctor's schedule was available and affordable.

I left the office and dialed Dr. Galland's number on my way home. His secretary answered and told me his schedule was booked for the month of August. My shoulders slumped in disappointment. I asked for the earliest availability. She was silent as she searched through his calendar. All of a sudden, her tone changed. "Wait, a patient canceled their appointment this morning. It's in two weeks. Do you want that?"

Two weeks was doable—a miracle. I snagged it.

We discussed the consultation fee; hearing the cost of $800 made my chest tighten. He was another out-of-network doctor. Not surprised by that news, I agreed to the amount without Jeff's approval. I gave her my information and she told me to expect paperwork in the mail in a few days. They wanted all the information filled out before I arrived at my consultation.

I updated my mother and shared my financial concerns. She insisted on calling a relative for another option. "We have a great doctor in the family who works at the Cleveland Clinic. Let's see who he suggests."

I needed her to slow down. I believed this doctor was my last chance.

"Just wait! My consultation is in two weeks. If nothing comes from that, then fine, you can call."

"Deal, but this time I'm going with you. I have my own questions for this doctor."

A week later, I received the package of forms from the new doctor's office. I was overwhelmed by the amount of paperwork: fifteen pages, some double-sided. I procrastinated and placed the packet on the kitchen counter. Every time I passed through the kitchen, I stared at those forms, dreading the task.

It was late Friday night, a weekend away from my consultation, and everyone was asleep in the house but me. I tossed and turned, worried about my girls' newest adventure. Abby and Jolie were leaving early the next morning for an overnight experience at their cousins' sleep away camp. We wanted to make sure they liked it before we made a final decision on whether or not to send them the following summer. I worried about homesickness during their first summer at camp—though perhaps I was simply more worried about missing them. The truth is the girls were more concerned about my strength, and my ability to catch them when they would jump into my arms on visiting day.

I wasn't sleeping anytime soon, distracted by Jeff's snoring. I left the bedroom and headed for the den. As I passed through the kitchen, I stopped, grabbed a pen and the doctor's paperwork. I had procrastinated long enough. I sat down on the couch and plowed through the first few pages. As I provided the necessary details to my chronic illness, I got emotional, taking stock of the inordinate amount of time and money I had spent searching for a diagnosis. It had taken more than a year of my life, and I was saddened by how much my family had suffered. I was frightened I might never get an answer, acknowledging the possibility of accepting this current state forever. I pushed the remainder of the packet aside and opened my laptop.

I stared at the blank screen of a Microsoft Word document and began typing without purpose or thought—just raw emotion pouring out of me. I filled ten pages, three hours after I typed my first word. I sighed with relief, closed the laptop and finished the rest of the packet.

I met my mother in front of Dr. Galland's office ten minutes before my appointment. She was full of pep and smiles, ever hopeful for a diagnosis. She had not yet experienced the disappointment from the many consultations I already had. We rode the elevator to the eighth floor and checked in. The waiting room seated a maximum of six people and seemed crowded. I knew it would be a while before my name was called. My mother read her book while I pulled off the strands of Buddy's hair from the cheap black sundress I wore most days.

I leaned my head against the wall but hesitated to shut my eyes. "Rest if your eyes burn," my mother whispered. "I'll wake you when it's our turn." I was glad she came.

I woke up startled when my mother tapped my shoulder. "He's ready for us."

We sat on the couch next to each other in his office, face to face with two different doctors. Dr. Galland introduced himself and his colleague, who asked permission to sit in on our appointment. I agreed with the notion that the more doctors who listened to my mysterious diagnosis, the better chance I had of finding an answer. I handed over my records.

I was impressed with the doctor's soft-spoken demeanor, especially after learning he had published four books, covering new scientific research relating to the immune system and weight loss, the power of healing oneself through integrative wellness and sound nutrition. I hoped he was a good speed-reader, watching him race through my files. Every few seconds, he tossed a handful of papers into the garbage and shared a few results with his colleague. The eighty sheets of test results I savored now looked rather slim and meaningless, calling attention to my fax machine fiasco at Staples.

He closed my file, looked up and wanted to hear my story. He pulled out his pad. "Start at the beginning—just before you got sick."

I recapped the months of my marathon training, my size two physique and the disappearance of my period. "Three weeks after the half-marathon, we brought a Golden Retriever puppy home."

He cut me off, looking over the tip of his glasses and asked, "You got a dog?"

I nodded.

"You have chronic giardiasis," he said with more confidence than any other doctor I had met. I was amazed that he diagnosed my illness within the first ten minutes of our appointment.

"My dog had giardia, but I've tested negative for this parasite a handful of times and been told that I don't have it, so how could it be?"

He explained that most stool tests are only fifty percent foolproof and there was only one doctor in the city whose test results he trusted. I was to make an appointment with that parasitologist and confirm this diagnosis. My mother grabbed my hand, squeezing it tightly. I glanced at her and caught the smile on her face, clinging to a glimmer of hope.

A few minutes later, while being examined, he sympathized with all my complaints. It seemed as if he understood more than anyone else. He injected vitamin B12 into my arm to help with the fatigue. If my energy improved over the next few days, he offered a prescription as long as I agreed to give myself a shot at home. At this point, I'd do anything for some energy on a daily basis. I asked how he diagnosed my case so quickly.

"You have a basketball-shaped belly." I wondered why he was the only doctor who described my stomach that way. He noticed the quizzical look on my face and continued, "I also had giardia for five months and my belly was the same shape."

I gasped. Could it be I had finally found the person who not only would help me, but had actually walked the same path, belly and all? Now he seemed to be in perfect health. He was thin and had a flat stomach. I believed I had met my last and final doctor.

We discussed my next steps, the possibility of a longer recovery and duration of weight loss. He wasn't sure what damage the parasite caused over the last fourteen months. He wanted to confirm giardia immediately and stop the steroids slowly, lowering the dose.

"Hormones can accelerate the infection." Apparently, steroids had made my situation worse. At this point, I didn't need to hear the scientific explanation behind his comment. I was perfectly content with just a diagnosis.

My mother shrieked and jumped up off the couch, hugging the doctor, relieved that my nightmare had ended. I laughed, brushing off her enthusiasm, even though I wanted to get up and dance. After all this time, I needed to believe all of this was true.

I called Jeff as we exited the building, while my mom dialed my dad. I rambled on about chronic giardiasis and couldn't wait for Jeff to partake in our excitement.

He hesitated, questioning the diagnosis.

"I don't want you to get your hopes up because if he's wrong, you'll be devastated again." I felt sucker-punched. It was one thing for me to harbor that secret doubt, but I expected Jeff to be as elated as my mother. I needed him to believe in this doctor and his word so that indeed, it could be true. I imagined Jeff wanted nothing more than for me to return to the woman he married, but now I wasn't so sure. Other than my recent breakdown in our bedroom, where we only discussed my feelings, Jeff didn't let on how he was feeling, but I knew he was also scared.

"Trust me. This time it's the real deal and as soon as the parasitologist confirms my diagnosis, I'll be able to start the antibiotics."

I explained a few more details, hoping he'd change opinions.

"I'll believe it when I see it," he said.

I understood the root of Jeff's skepticism. We had tried many times to get pregnant before the girls, and I recognized that same caution in his voice—as though I had just told him I was pregnant with not just one baby, but two. I hoped Jeff would see the light soon.

I hung up the phone and hugged my mother. If she hadn't been there, maybe I would have also doubted the diagnosis. I wondered if our friends and family thought I had been crying wolf for fourteen months, but I was back to the very first thing I suggested when I asked that first doctor, "I have a puppy who has giardia. Do you think I could have it, too?"

Between expensive doctor consultations, hospital visits, acupuncture treatments, medications and the many herbal supplements, it had cost us about $35,000 out-of-pocket just to get to this point. In a few short days, I'd be taking the same medication Buddy took over a year ago—a simple antibiotic. Every time I'd look at him, I couldn't help but think I wouldn't be in this situation if we never brought him home—and I was certain he was not my Buddy.

CHAPTER
17

DR. CAHILL, THE PARASITOLOGIST, was in his early seventies and had studied tropical medicine while working for decades with the United Nations and many third world countries. I sat in his office, discussing the history of my health. After I recapped the last fourteen months, he seemed confident with Dr. Galland's diagnosis.

A few minutes later, we were in the examination room, testing for giardia. I expected a take-home stool kit like the previous doctors provided. Instead, I anxiously watched as he jellied up a long white scope that was moments away from scraping the inside of my anal walls.

Evidently, a person infected with giardia doesn't expel cysts every time they go to the bathroom. As he completed the specimen and handed over a box of tissues, he explained that there are two types of giardia: the active form, which exists in the gut of an infected person, or the inactive cyst form, which can remain dormant in the environment for several months.

He explained in further details the medical terms. Though it all sounded like gibberish to me, I spent time researching his publications and later understood the situation. According to an online medical dictionary, once cysts were ingested, the acid in my stomach broke them down, causing the active parasite to be released into my body. The parasite attached to the lining of my small intestines, multiplied, then traveled into the fecal stream. Once the feces become dry, the parasites form cysts again, and over time, leave the body through bowel movements.

After fourteen months learning my body's anatomy, I still needed the basic explanation. Dr. Cahill saw the perplexed look on my face. "In other words, giardia attaches to the villi and immobilizes that part of the body. It then stimulates inflammation and the inflammation interferes with food absorption. Eventually, the infection causes food malabsorption and havoc in your digestive tract, not to mention other parts of the body."

A light went on. "That would explain why I found whole pieces of food in my stool—the bud, leaf and partial stem of broccoli rabe!" I sat up for the blood test and changed topics, hoping he'd have answers to my weight gain. "Why do most people have diarrhea from parasites and lose weight, but the opposite happened to me?"

"We know there's a correlation between the condition of one's immune system and the severity of their symptoms. A person with a compromised immune system may not be able to fight off this infection as easily as someone in great health," he said, waiting for my blood to fill the vial.

I sat quietly, mulling over his comments as he yanked the rubber band from my arm and pulled out the needle. That was the second time a doctor used the word 'compromised'. Dr. Galland referred to it when I questioned the timeframe of my recovery, and now Dr. Cahill implied that it was connected to my symptoms.

When he left the room, I considered what my health condition was prior to bringing Buddy home. Clearly I thought I was in good shape based on my appearance and the fact that I could run half marathons. Eight months ago, my acupuncturist Chris mentioned how years of my daily behaviors attributed to the demise of my immune system. Finally, it sunk in. I had played a huge role in my own perfect storm. On the outside, I had looked physically fit but inside, I was a mess and the giardia was the last nail towards self-detonation.

The doctor recommended that Jeff get tested as well.

"I've seen it a handful of times where unknowingly, couples continuously infect each other from oral sex. Both spouses need to be checked or they'll never get rid of it."

Even though Jeff showed no symptoms, I refused to be that couple. There was no way we could have infected each other, I thought, realizing how little intimacy we shared since all of this happened. By the time I left his office, I scheduled Jeff for his own scraping the next day.

Twenty-four hours after my exam, I sat on the couch with the phone in hand, anxiously awaiting my results—hoping to solve a fourteen-month mystery. Buddy rested his snout on my feet, hoping to get attention. I felt butterflies inside my distended belly. It didn't matter that I believed in this diagnosis, I needed confirmation that my search was finally over.

My anxiety reminded me of my two-year struggle with infertility. I had spent countless hours longing to experience 'the pregnant belly' and now, I'd do anything to get rid of it. With the girls at day camp and Jeff at work, I dialed Dr. Cahill's office—ready to reclaim my life.

Buddy changed positions and rested his snout on my lap. I leaned forward and braced myself, hearing the nurse's voice.

"The doctor found cysts of giardia in your specimen. You have the parasite."

I was stunned and relieved at the same time, confident my nightmare had just ended. My eyes shut as I received this closure and a grin spread across my face. The death sentence that brought me to my knees quickly vanished, and all I needed now was a course of antibiotics.

"You should call Dr. Galland's office later today for the prescription. You'll need to be retested two weeks after you finished the antibiotics."

I eagerly scheduled my next scraping.

My hands shook as I stared at the phone and listened to a dial tone, distinctly recalling the same surge of relief when I heard a nurse tell me, "you're pregnant." I was ecstatic, reveling in my news, not knowing whom to call first—Jeff, my mother or the veterinarian.

Buddy moved his head towards my face, looking at me with the same droopy eyes that once warmed my heart. As soon as I caught a glimpse of his saliva-bubbled tongue, I backed away, disgusted. I called the vet and got an appointment for him the next day. I needed proof that Buddy was clean before I ever touched him again.

Jeff got his results the next day. I was floored to learn he had tested positive for giardia. I shouldn't have been surprised, considering transmission between couples, but it seemed so impossible for us that I thought I had heard him wrong.

"Really?" I asked, wondering why Jeff's body hadn't changed one bit.

"I also have to get rechecked in two weeks," he said with gravity in his tone.

Our conversation immediately returned to finances; each test would cost $395. Jeff was panicking for all the right reasons, but I refused to address his concerns.

"I need to call Dr. Galland. I'll talk to you later."

During the afternoon, I rested on the couch, waiting for a call from the doctor. My resentments grew the more I fixated on the fact that Jeff had not gained weight or experienced any of my symptoms. I sat around wallowing in self-pity and agonizing over my past behaviors, all the while aware that I was the one who weakened my own immune system. Jeff never ran miles in the rain when he was sick. He took better care of himself than I had and for that reason alone, his body wasn't compromised and was able to fight the infection. I only felt worse realizing my stupidity was the sole reason for our additional financial stress.

Dr. Galland prescribed antibiotics for our entire family because the likelihood that the infection could have spread within our household was extremely high. Apparently, I ingested a microscopic speckle after cleaning one of Buddy's "chocolate messes," even after I washed my hands. Knowing I handled the girls' food over the last fourteen months, the doctor questioned if they were asymptomatic like their father. As far as I knew, they were.

I wished I had followed the same protocol that I taught them to wash hands while singing 'Happy Birthday,' twice. Either way, it was too late. There was no way to avoid six days of grueling battles, crushing pills into powder and sprinkling it into Abby's and Jolie's favorite foods, praying it all went down.

Alinia, the prescribed antibiotic, had side effects. The pill was rather large to ingest, left an awful metal taste in our mouths, made everyone tired and caused a lot of stomach pain. Jeff and I took 500 milligrams twice a day, while the girls were given half that dosage, once a day. My chest tightened every time they complained and I blamed Buddy, which only made the girls more upset.

Jolie raced to Buddy's side. "That's so mean, mom. He's just a puppy." She giggled as his wet tongue slid across her cheeks, then, moved to the tips of her fingers. The possibility of infection never crossed her mind, or left mine.

"Great Jo, now go wash your face and hands." Anytime he licked Jeff or the girls, I cringed and found myself at the veterinarian's office the next day.

Buddy's stool sample was clean. I inquired further, since many of my own samples were invalid. Ironically, the vet claimed the test for animals was highly sensitive and therefore, accurate—way more accurate than the tests given to people. If there wasn't something wrong with this, I wasn't sure what else I would discover about the medical community in regard to giardia that wouldn't completely blow my mind.

"If anything, we find most results are false positive, not negative," he said.

I knew that giardia cysts lived for several months in cool, wet conditions and those same cysts were also found on dog's hair from the constant licking of their genitals.

"Is it possible that touching Buddy may transfer giardia?" I asked.

In short, the answer was yes, and my imagination ran amok with all the places we'd been where he could have received a transmission: dog parks, overnight kennels, lakes, street puddles and even my own backyard. Where was it safe for Buddy to roam? Was it safe for us? I imagined newspaper headlines: *Forget The Bubble Boy: Meet The Bubble Buddy.*

"Too bad I didn't know all this when we got Buddy, I would have worn gloves and a face mask," I told the vet.

"I wish you told me you were sick. I've seen this happen with other clients of mine."

Buddy raised his front paw and placed it on the vet's lap, stealing his attention.

"I could have told you it was giardia," he said, shaking his head.

My eyes widened. We spent $35,000 on top-notch doctors and the whole time the veterinarian could have diagnosed my condition for $65. It was time to face the facts. Having Buddy had only contributed to our woes. It was time to consider getting rid of him.

I questioned Buddy's future and imagined announcing his departure to the girls: Jolie in tears, wrapping her arms around Buddy's neck, declaring, "He's our family! It's not fair," while Jeff stood by my side in silence, displaying the same look of disappointment as the rest of them.

I was ashamed to think this, but the veterinarian gave me more reasons to stop and consider what the hell I was doing with our dog. It made no sense to keep him when he made me sick, and it was possible I could get giardia again, but I couldn't quite wrap my head around giving him away. The girls would never forgive me; I had already disappointed them enough.

Two weeks later, after the antibiotics worked their magic, I received word from Dr. Cahill's office that I tested negative for giardia. I was eager to continue Dr. Galland's protocol and use the antibiotic Fluconazole for fourteen days, hoping to rid my gut of yeast overgrowth until I could reduce the dosage of steroids by half. I also started other natural supplements to rebuild my adrenal glands, coat my stomach lining, digest my food, ease the constipation and support my immune system. He offered a prescription of vitamin B12 shots after I reported a slight increase of energy. I jumped at the opportunity, hoping to expedite my recovery.

After years of infertility shots, I assumed I'd be comfortable giving myself a shot until the moment I stood in my kitchen, needle in hand, and panicked. I phoned Jeff at work and begged him to come home. Instead, he suggested speakerphone in order to free up my hands while he attempted to talk me through it, directing our conversation towards sex. Unfortunately, I neglected to mention that the cleaning ladies had arrived and noticed them in the background, so I quickly jabbed the needle into my thigh, avoiding further embarrassment. When I told him, he belted out in laughter. That was the last time I asked for a pep talk.

Content with Dr. Galland's regimen, I shared the diagnosis with the medical team. They appreciated the update and wished me well. While it was nice to spend less time in each of their offices, I missed the kinship I received from those specialists. I had grown fond of their support, discussions and the many lessons I learned. They had become a huge part of my daily life and knew more about my current issues than my friends; now however, I placed my recovery in the hands of one doctor. I really believed I was at the end of my search.

By the middle of October 2009, I was back in Dr. Galland's office for the third follow-up appointment. My stomach was still very distended, despite having stopped the steroids and continuing a meticulous diet, avoiding: gluten, soy, dairy, eggs, certain beans and peanuts. At my last consultation, the doctor added a few more supplements to my protocol, trying to jumpstart my metabolism, which made no difference other than crowding my kitchen counter-top. I was anxious for new suggestions that worked.

While I waited in the reception area, I got a call from our cleaning lady. I figured she needed the garage code since that's the only time she had ever called me in the past. We usually text each other so when we spoke, the connection was unclear.

She sounded out of breath and shouted, "Buddy's outside and we can't get him back in the house."

My mouth dropped open. Buddy had never been off leash on our front property. He was only allowed in our fenced-in backyard. She explained how the inside door to the garage wasn't shut all the way and how he escaped while one of them was throwing out the garbage.

I was in the city, at least forty-five minutes from home.

I panicked.

"Are you kidding me? You have to get him back."

I insisted they rush to the fridge and take a fistful of Trader Joe's diced white meat chicken since Buddy never missed an opportunity to snack. I figured once they got close enough, one of the women could grab his collar.

"Do whatever you have to and call me as soon as you have him."

I called Jeff and freaked out. He rambled on about how irresponsible it was of the cleaning ladies.

"Seriously?" I asked. "Just call and help her!"

My mind raced while I waited by the phone, confronting the possibility of life without Buddy. At this point, for all I knew he could be hit by a car. My hands trembled, imagining all the moments I took for granted. I wished I could take back every thought I had about giving him away, as I was encouraged to do by many friends and acquaintances when they learned of my diagnosis. I loathed this suggestion, but I hated that people actually said what I had thought. Of course, getting rid of the source of the problem, Buddy, seemed totally logical but it wasn't entirely his fault. I was part of the problem, too, and had made it worse by compromising my own immune system. As much as I wanted to avoid taking another dose of harsh medicine, or any medicine at all, I had to accept my role in creating this whole situation.

Sitting there sobered by the reality that this was the day I might lose Buddy for good, I realized I could never give him away because we believed he made me sick. Just as I could never picture my world without the girls, I could not imagine our lives without Buddy. He was a part of our family, and all I wanted was for him to return home safe and sound.

I called Jeff, desperate for an update. While on the phone, my neighbor called me.

"Are you aware there are four women chasing your dog up the block?"

When I heard my cleaning lady's voice, I calmed down a bit, relieved to learn that Buddy was on a leash and headed back to my house. I wondered if this would have happened had I kept up with Buddy's intensive training, but had no time to think clearly at the doctor's office. I had to stay focused on the task at hand: clearly articulating recent issues.

When I was finally called to Dr. Galland's office, I pulled out a list of topics to discuss. I had written these questions ahead of time, so that I didn't forget anything during the appointment. After the Buddy escape, my mind was reeling, and I was grateful for my notes—though alarmed at the doctor's response.

Dr. Galland wasn't satisfied with my progress either. Apparently, some of my symptoms should have subsided by now. He prescribed 500 milligrams of Metronidazole, another antibiotic to be taken three times per day. He explained that it was not easy to rid the body of giardia, especially when the parasite thrived inside for long periods of time. He switched medications, knowing giardia becomes resistant against each antibiotic. He mentioned the possibility that the cysts could keep re-infecting me. I was eager to move beyond this phase and lose the weight. He requested another visit to

Dr. Cahill's office, two weeks after I finished the latest round of medication. He couldn't treat my other symptoms until I was giardiafree. I could hardly believe what I had heard. His announcement sounded distant, floating above me in that office. The road to my recovery was far from over. I had no idea how long it would take to lose the weight or if it was even still possible. If giardia had become my leash, I wanted some lessons from Buddy on mastering my great escape.

The drive home from the city seemed endless. My shoulders tightened from guilt while dwelling on Buddy's safety. Now, I even considered going back to basics, crating him when leaving the house or gating him in the kitchen as a way to avoid future getaways. I gripped the steering wheel harder at the thought of taking Buddy's freedom away when I was the one who cut his training short. No wonder he wasn't able to obey all commands.

I recalled the time when Abby was five years old and I lost her in Bed, Bath and Beyond. I let go of the girls' hands, scanning the back of the shelves for a certain pattern of window treatments, while keeping track of my children's chitchat until there was silence. I felt a flush of nerves explode through my body, knowing something was wrong. I spun around to find only Jolie standing by my side. Frightened that my worst fear was becoming my reality, I grabbed Jolie's hand, yanking her through every aisle, shouting Abby's name. I stopped customers nearby, hoping they saw a child matching my description but no one saw her. Panicked that she was gone, tears blurred my vision. My heart pounded and blood flushed my face. Then I heard the intercom repeat my name, asking me to report to customer service. We ran to the front of the store, where Abby stood next to the manager, holding her hand. I dropped to my knees and hugged her tightly, never wanting our embrace to end. When she couldn't find us, Abby told me she went for help at the front desk. I grabbed her cheeks with both my hands and smiled with pride, knowing she followed my directions. I wished I had spent the same amount of time teaching Buddy as I had with the girls, but I hadn't, so I couldn't expect him to be as well-behaved. It wasn't fair to punish him as a result. Now, I only wanted to see him and hug him too.

I pulled into my driveway and pressed the garage door opener. When I entered the house shouting Buddy's name, he was anxiously waiting at the door. I bent down, throwing my arms around his neck. He immediately sat up, kept eye contact with me and lifted his front paw, which landed on my thigh. Buddy followed my every move until I was situated on the den couch where he lay by my feet.

At one point, he sat up and rested his snout on my knees, looking for attention. I smiled at him, scratching the top of his head. After another day of disappointments and unanswered questions, I should have been anything but content. As I held his gaze, he raised his paw and rested it on my knee. A few minutes later, I stood up from the couch and grabbed a few pillows, while Buddy watched me carefully. I switched spots and lay on the floor, wanting to show him more affection.

"Come here, Boo," I said, patting a spot on the den carpet. He trotted over and snuggled next to me, granting my once great wish to have a big and loyal dog. We spent the next hour waiting for the girls while I petted him. All my problems seemed to fade away while having this loving dog by my side. Despite how much weight I gained or lost—God willing—there was no chance in hell I'd ever get rid of Buddy.

A month later, I was elated when I tested negative for giardia. During the next visit, Dr. Galland prescribed ten days of Itraconazole, hoping to clear up any lingering yeast overgrowth. While there, he reminded me that inflamed areas in the body block communication between cells and their receptor sites, causing those systems to disconnect. Without communication amongst these systems, my body wouldn't work well. He gave me two different take-home kits: one provided the latest twenty-four hour reading of my cortisol levels and the other tested my intestinal permeability. I concluded that my digestive tract was compromised from the parasite, stress, toxins, medications and nutrient deficiencies, causing Leaky Gut.

I had never heard of this test and asked for more clarification. Apparently, when the intestine is inflamed, this causes the intestinal lining to become hyperpermeable to large molecules. When this occurs, these molecules penetrate the intestine wall and stimulate a more aggressive immune response. The inflamed cells may also lose the ability to produce certain enzymes, resulting in malnutrition and food sensitivities. In addition to leaky gut, malnutrition and food sensitivities, intestinal giardiasis is also associated with an overgrowth of yeast and bacteria in the small intestine. The inflammation resulting from giardiasis in about 30-50% of cases allows the yeast and bacteria to proliferate and contribute to inflammation. It's a vicious cycle.

Dr. Galland also drew an extensive panel of blood to test for the many strains of Lyme Disease, other nutritional deficiencies, auto-immune diseases as well as the food allergen test. I was overwhelmed again. Lyme Disease? Seriously? After all of this? I refused to believe that I had anything else in my body other than giardia. I could not handle knowing that we had only knocked down one pin in the bowling alley. The list went on. He encouraged me to have my home checked for mold. Mold? He wanted to pinpoint every system that could have been compromised by living with Chronic Giardiasis.

I returned from my doctor's appointment minutes before the girls were dismissed from school. It rained most of the day, causing heavy traffic on the drive home. By the time we entered the garage, Abby realized she had forgotten her math homework. I glanced through the rearview mirror, noticing the disappointment on her face. She knew I was exhausted from the doctor's appointment and needed to rest. They, too, felt burdened by my agitation.

Jolie was hungry and asked to grab a snack from the pantry before we drove back to the school.

"Make sure to close the door behind you since Buddy's not gated anymore," I said as she ran inside the house. Abby remained quiet in the back seat so I turned around and faced her.

"Sweetie, it's not a big deal. Please don't think twice about it," I said, grateful to provide some comfort and endurance. I would survive driving back to the school.

Within seconds, Jolie hopped back into the car, closing the garage door behind us, but by the time we returned home again and parked in the garage, Abby hollered, "Mom, Buddy's out!"

I slammed the passenger door, stepping inches from the SUV trunk. "Are you serious?" I asked, flinching over what I was about to witness. I turned around and spotted him on the driveway, inches from the garage door and regretted that I hadn't already closed the outside door before I left the car. We stood frozen, as our eyes were fixated on one another, playing an intense game of chicken. The lack of dog training came back to haunt me.

I softly said, "Quick, go get his leash and the Trader Joe's Chicken from the fridge," while maintaining eye contact. As soon as Abby returned, Buddy ran off, galloping between the front lawn and driveway, making what looked like large figure eights. I grabbed everything from Abby's hands and darted toward his direction, causing him to run further. He stopped in the middle of the street. I worried Buddy would be struck by a car speeding around the bend. I shouted, waving the carton of his favorite food, "You want this Buddy? Then, come," but he didn't budge. Jolie stood on the front porch and watched as I sprinted towards him, assuming he'd at least get out of the street. He only scampered further down the hill. I stood on my front property wet, cold and without a jacket, wearing rubber rain boots that covered my calves. I was in no shape to run and shouted, "Buddy, come!" He stopped in his tracks about three homes down. I hollered again but he refused to come. I was exhausted and needed to sit down for a moment. I turned in Jolie's direction when I saw the look on her pale face.

"Mom, please don't give up on him." Jolie cried, reminding me of my responsibility as Buddy's "mother." I wished I had accomplished this one simple command at the beginning.

I took a deep breath and spun around and leapt from property to property, chasing him. Buddy raced towards a neighbor's boxer out for a stroll. Within seconds, they were in the street, barking and jumping on top of each other. While the boxer was on a leash, I was afraid to intervene, remembering the moment I was bitten on the leg by a small dog at my parents' friend's house. I stood paralyzed in the street.

"Give me your leash," the owner said, grabbing Buddy's leash from me and quickly attaching it to his collar. I admired how her dog obeyed her every word. She handed over Buddy's leash. I yanked him away, apologizing and thanking her immensely. On my way home, I didn't speak, infuriated that I'd lost control over Buddy because of giardia and god knows whatever else. I tossed him into the crate for a time out and called Jeff, knowing how the cleaning ladies must have felt. This time, however, there was no incident too terrible to make me ever think about giving him away. Buddy, crazy figure-eight maker and all, was home for good.

By late November 2009, eighteen months of exhaustion finally subsided, thanks to the daily injections of vitamin B12. While I wasn't ready for marathons, I drove carpools, hosted play dates, spent quality time with my girls and returned to the gym, where I started Pilates classes twice a week. My family appreciated my presence and the increased responsibility I reclaimed around the household, picking up the slack that I had continuously piled onto Jeff.

My life resembled a sense of normalcy—other than forty extra pounds I was carrying and a stack of medical bills that our health insurance never covered. This had become our new normal. Jeff owned a small business and paid a $12,000 annual medical insurance premium, which included a $5,000 deductible per individual or $10,000 deductible as a family. Somehow the many procedures and tests had not qualified; only some expenses were allotted toward our deductible.

Prior to my condition, our annual medical expenses were minimal because we stayed within network, but after so many out of network specialists, we received almost no reimbursements. I was burdened with guilt and stopped the acupuncture sessions, doctor consultations, laboratory and hospital tests, but still had to pay for the constant refills of supplements, follow-up visits to doctors, blood work and take-home tests.

The supplements were some of the biggest expenses. Most bottles provided enough pills to last for only two weeks, and they cost between thirty to fifty dollars each. I feared a relapse and adhered to the doctor's regimen even though my metabolism had stabilized. Once my bowels regulated, the intense pressure around my stomach only decreased slightly but left my skin flabby.

During my next appointment in December 2009, Dr. Galland reviewed every test result and requested I stop all the supplements but two bottles. He focused on supporting my adrenal glands and promoting healthy cell membrane by maximizing the fuel in my mitochondria—the energy source of the body. It seemed my immune system showed some improvement based on a few levels that returned to a normal range. As he scanned further, he pointed out other levels that appeared abnormal, testing positive for Epstein-Barr. He questioned whether the antibody panel was active, recent or from an old infection

Epstein-Barr? I had no idea what this was but it didn't sound good. No disease named after a person ever sounded good. Parkinson's. Lou Gehrig's. Lyme. Where was all this going? I felt the heat of a newflame of hell flaring on the horizon. I thought I was about to reclaim my life and finally get a handle on our expenses, but I was wrong.

It became clear that I had only caught a glimpse of what my recovery truly entailed. I longed for my acupuncturist's lengthy explanations until I understood each subject. Now, I was left to my own edification and worried these latest findings would prolong my healing and weight loss even further. I questioned the tests' validity and next steps of my protocol.

Dr. Galland looked up at me while flipping the page and calmly responded, "We'll keep an eye on those markers but I'm not too concerned. They're likely to be false positive." He reminded me that by age thirty-eight, most patients have had antibodies to the Epstein-Barr virus. He didn't think the result was valid and moved to the next set.

"You fell within reference range but on the outside of the Intestinal Permeability test." He wasn't surprised and switched my current probiotics. I stayed quiet while absorbing more explanations. He handed me a copy of a fifteen-page food allergen report that listed foods by categories. I assumed from a previous test done by Chris that gluten, soy, dairy, peanuts, eggs and a few type of beans appeared on this list but fretted there would be even more foods to avoid on this new list. While he spoke, I quickly scanned the pages, as if I had been given my children's class lists for the first time, only in this case, praying for the opposite results—names of foods I didn't recognize. I was relieved to see that bananas, tuna, cilantro and baker's/brewer's yeast were added to the list. Life without those foods seemed doable. I was becoming a professional at this part, at least.

I assumed I was in the clear until I reached the last three pages of the packet where I found another list of foods categorized under the heading, Intestinal Barrier Assessment. I shuddered, seeing many of my favorite foods: chicken, shrimp, apples, and oranges. Even if I forced myself to eat beef and pork, I couldn't because those were on the list, too.

"What's the difference between the two lists and which do I have to follow?" I asked, worried his answer was both.

Apparently, these tests looked at two different types of antibodies against foods. The first set listed IGE allergic antibodies, which included foods to which my body was previously exposed. The allergic reaction is caused from a leaky gut versus the food itself. The second list included IGG antibodies. High levels of IGG would indicate a leaky gut—and further evidence that my immune system was taxed. I was devastated by this news and aggravated that I had to seek new options.

"It's not easy to completely change your diet overnight but you'll have to find foods that aren't on this list," he sympathized.

As he wrote down directions to my latest protocol, I begged for additional assistance with my metabolism. Clearly, cutting out more foods wasn't helping. I asked to increase my thyroid medication, hoping a higher dose would increase communication between cells. Worst case, I'd end up with hyperthyroidism and be granted symptoms such as extreme weight loss, ignoring all the other negative side effects. He refused, worried that even 120 milligrams was already too high, potentially causing future cardiovascular issues, among other problems. He stopped mid-sentence, sat quietly for a moment and considered other options, sensing my frustration.

He offered a medication typically given to diabetics called Bromocriptine, sharing two examples of patients who had lost weight as a result. I heard the words 'weight loss' and jumped at the chance to be his next guinea pig. He started me on the lowest dosage and hoped to slowly increase it over the next four weeks or until my body became intolerant. He opened the door and walked me to the reception area, reminding me of the potential side effects and added, "If you feel faint, nauseated or even light headed, call my office."

On my way home from the city, I called my mother with an update, brushing through topics, wondering if what I said made any sense. I was dreading friends' phone calls, knowing very well I couldn't handle the amount of questions they would ask. Worst of all, I feared the escalating costs. I wondered if there would be enough time to heal my body before I threatened my family's future financial stability. My head ached from all that was still unknown.

A month on Bromocryptine was all I could tolerate. I experienced every symptom the doctor mentioned, yet nothing changed with my weight. My fluctuating hormone levels were contributing to inflammation on a cyclic basis. Dr. Galland tried everything to help me, but hormones weren't his specialty. During my last appointment in January, he recommended a holistic gynecologist experienced in hormonal imbalances. I was extremely apprehensive to leave the doctor who diagnosed my condition and start with a new specialist who could address my hormone issues. It was clear that if I wanted to recover, I had to incur additional costs, start from scratch, and dump more half-used bottles of supplements for another regimen.

CHAPTER
18

APPROACHED HOLISTIC and Functional Medicine with an open mind. I thought I was fairly receptive to the theories suggested so far until I passed the baton to my next potential healer. I had left a doctor on Fifth Avenue who wore a crisp suit and tie and headed for the suburbs. Now, I sat across from a new doctor who wore a basic button down shirt, outdated jeans and sported a ponytail which held what little remained of his white hair.

I had been used to defending a doctor's protocol of mixing prescribed medications with a combination of natural supplements. However, it was a challenge to accept a practice that relied entirely on herbal remedies. While I knew this recommendation was from a reliable source, I felt as if I had entered the twilight zone. In no time at all, I was leaving monthly appointments with lengthy shopping lists of supplements and a handful of take-home

kits. I was assigned to test my saliva for cell weakness associated
with my metabolism, and to complete a urine analysis test for
heavy metal toxins and acid levels.

The treatment started with a twenty-eight day detoxification
cleanse, alleviating intestinal inflammation and helping with leptin
resistance, a hormone associated with excess weight caused by
impaired cell communication from the pituitary gland. I took a
variety of supplements such as DHEA, Conjugated Linolenic
Acid, Acetyl L Carnitine, B6 Phosphate and CoQ10.

I combined Estrium powder with measured flaxseed and fish
oils into a daily shake as a second detox, focusing on my estrogen
metabolism. Then I added Estrodim pills into the regimen once
the second detox was completed. I ingested 50,000 units of vitamin
D in liquid form weekly, extended over a twelve-week period, and
drank tablespoons of watered-down apple cider vinegar before
every meal in addition to the supplements I continued from Dr.
Galland to support my immune system.

I even purchased essential oils used for holistic breast massaging
and was told it brought healing energy and health into my breast
tissue. I made castor oil packs using a cloth, towel, heating pad and
plastic sheet, stimulating lymphatic drainage around my abdomen
while following suggested meditation and visualization exercises.

Jeff assisted nightly with all the prep work while I lay down on
a plastic sheet, half naked with headphones on as he covered my
abdomen with the warm cloth that dripped of castor oil. Without
fail, he uttered a sinister laugh, like a mad scientist who prepared
a secret potion. And this was intimacy, I thought, baffled by the
regimen as well. I wasn't sure if I was grateful to experience a
moment of closeness with Jeff or embarrassed by the very protocol
that created it, knowing those moments were just about the only
time we ever genuinely laughed together. I tried tape recording one
follow-up appointment so that Jeff and my mother could finally

make sense of my test results. The only problem was that I pressed play instead of record.

By the end of winter 2010, I saw my acupuncturist weekly. I needed reassurance that this doctor wasn't a huge waste of time, effort and money. I knew with Chris's knowledge and attentiveness, he'd be able to decipher between the recent results and my interpretations of them, plus concentrate on my biggest frustration —the lack of weight loss. He added a handful of supplements once I showed more signs of increased energy. As each system healed and became more balanced, my chances of losing the weight seemed greater. I emailed the doctor a complete list of supplements, hoping to eliminate some, but the list kept growing.

By the middle of March, the doctor added a few rounds of Chelation Therapy to my protocol, convinced my heavy metal count was still too high and interfered with cellular function. He also introduced Trialkali powder and baths taken in Epsom salts, reducing high acid levels in my body. At this point, I could barely absorb any new concepts and disregarded further analysis. When Chris suggested more blood be drawn to test interleukin markers showing autoimmune inflammation, I proceeded, despite the out-of-pocket expense.

My digestive enzymes increased from one bottle to three, helping me to break down food particles: proteins, carbohydrates, fats and sugars that converted into nutrients my pancreas could absorb. I also tried two different bottles of supplements, wondering if Hypoglycemia or Insulin Resistance was an issue for me. My frequent complaints of lightheadedness in early mornings and late afternoons were an indication that my body wasn't processing sugar correctly. Soon, I was taking more than 132 pills per day, leaving me with little appetite for food. My family watched as my snack-sized Ziploc bags grew into sandwich-sized, holding over forty pills at each meal.

I charged more than $400 weekly for these supplements, praying the credit cards hadn't hit their limit. It was only a matter of time before the next bout with Jeff. Our arguments became more frequent, and I found myself hiding from him especially in the evenings when he paid the bills. It had been over a year and a half since we sat together on our bathroom floor when I agreed not to give up on 'us.' At this point, the finances were his burden and getting a diagnosis was mine. While I knew our finances were hurting, the only energy I could muster was directed towards my diagnosis. As a result, we were both miserable, stuck in a pile of quicksand while our marriage, vitality and finances sank.

That's when Chris suggested the concept of drinking freshly boiled herbs. I wouldn't have to refill the bottles of supplements as often, which would reduce the financial strains each week. I agreed immediately when he told me the herbs absorb into the system faster than pills. I would take anything in order to lose weight and lighten up the atmosphere around my household.

Every week, I spent $50 to lug home a gallon-sized bag of herbs, specifically chosen to boost my energy, metabolism and immune system. I dumped the bag into a large soup pot and boiled it for forty-five minutes, then covered one of my oversized square Tupperware containers with a jumbo strainer and dumped in the cloudy brown liquid, resembling sewer water. Once done, I put the Tupperware container into the refrigerator and drank eight ounce glasses twice a day, cringing with every gulp.

While my family ate a normal dinner, I nursed the glass of "mud" on an empty stomach. It was bad enough listening to my girls complain about the foul smell left in the kitchen after I cooked the herbs. They also apologized to their math tutor about it every week because they were embarrassed. The tutor was a good friend of mine and taught Kindergarten at a different elementary school in town. Her concern upon entering my house wasn't necessarily about the bad odor but how awful I felt. She'd look at me and insist on taking my girls to dinner after their session in order for me sleep in peace.

The commentary over the stench didn't stop with the girls. "You know we have the same piles of dirt in our own backyard that you can boil, at no charge," Jeff said, disgusted.

Sometimes I wondered if he thought I actually liked to drink "the mud" or ingest the supplements. Of course I wanted the same dietary habits as my family without worrying that my belly would balloon the next day, but this was the only option I was given. It was obvious that Jeff had enough of my hocus pocus experiments, and when the conversation came up about a spring break vacation, he lost his cool at the kitchen table.

He pointed his finger towards the granite countertop. "You see that kitchen counter over there covered by all your bottles? There's your family vacation fund." Our lifestyle was drastically changing each week. We searched for more ways to reduce our extravagant expenses and avoid the looming financial disaster. At the time, we thought one of the worst things to happen was withdrawing from our golf club. I never imagined that only a few years later we would be losing the house too. My perfect picture life was crumbling. One by one, pictures were falling off the wall of illusion, but it didn't matter if I had all the money in the world, no 'picture' could ever heal my health.

We were grateful for one blessed and timely gift in April. My parents took my sister's family and mine to the Dominican Republic to celebrate my dad's seventieth birthday during spring break. The only positive effect of my abundant credit card usage was the accumulation of bonus points, providing four free airline flights.

I was excited to go away and have some time to relax, but I wondered how I'd get through customs, schlepping more than twenty-five bottles of supplements, creams, and powders for the shakes—my "backyard dirt" according to Jeff. I imagined being pulled aside by airport security, frisked, arrested or worse, having all my supplies confiscated and left to repurchase.

After a lengthy argument, my husband refused to bring our blender, pot and strainer, but I was determined to follow the current regimen. I could not afford another setback.

While I shared the latest protocol with my family, nobody understood how it had taken over my life until we lived under the same roof again. When we arrived at the vacation house, I walked directly to the kitchen and searched for the necessary supplies to boil my herbs as everyone else unpacked their bags. I was thrilled to find a blender and pot. I still needed a strainer and sent my mother on a wild goose chase, asking the concierge, main kitchen and housekeeping, all of us lost in translation. Numerous times, she repeated, "A strainer," hoping someone spoke some English. "It's what you pour pasta into when it's ready." Frustrated by the confusion, her voice got louder. "Spaghetti," she enunciated. "Do you make spaghetti here?"

The following afternoon, she received word that the chef had found a strainer. When the doorbell rang, my mother answered and I heard her loud laugh. The strainer she held resembled something that belonged to my girls' American Girl Doll cookware set.

Regardless of the challenge, my mother found a way and boiled the herbs, reclaiming every last drop of brown liquid. I appreciated her determination, whether she agreed with the regimen or not. Throughout the rest of our vacation, I avoided further discussions about my condition, hating the questions. I just wanted to take my pills, drink my shakes and "mud," and move on with my day. I didn't want the added stress of family spying on my concoctions.

Over the next few months, I focused on my strict regimen and preparation for the girls' first overnight camp at the end of June. While we had cut back on all of our expenses, we did everything we could to make sure the girls could still go to camp. They were thrilled, trusting I was now strong enough to hold their little bodies when they jumped into my arms on visiting day. I appreciated my increased strength, exercise routine and the ability to enjoy many short distance runs, but was still sorely disappointed about my lack of weight loss.

For seven months, I had strictly followed the doctor's herbal remedies, spent thousands of additional dollars and ingested 132 pills per day, with only a ten-pound weight loss. I still had thirty more to lose. While most of my bloat dissipated, I refused another supplement—four weeks of Nystatin powder—especially after the latest course of yeast overgrowth treatment.

I had reached my limit toward this holistic approach after learning that my recent blood tests showed signs of overdosing on supplements and a high acidity level. The conundrum frustrated me. Why was my small body holding onto thirty extra pounds? I knew it was time for more expensive consultations and the probability of starting over once again.

The seasons felt like weeks. Spring morphed into the middle of the summer. It was evident I needed an endocrinologist, specializing in metabolism. At this point, the only qualification I required was for someone who produced results. I was less than thrilled to seek out more doctor referrals. Luckily, one of my best friends had a recommendation after spending time with this doctor. Apparently, he was listed in magazines as one of the top New York doctors. Next to his medical diploma from Yale University, photographs from his appearance on Good Morning America hung on his office walls. I was sold on his credentials and believed this was going to be my year of magical shrinking.

At the first consultation in August, I dumped a large shopping bag of supplements on the endocrinologist's desk. I sat quietly watching as he grabbed the different bottles, reading their ingredients with a perplexed expression. He insisted I stop most of the natural remedies except for a probiotic, claiming the amount of glycerin I ingested was more damaging than the benefits of the actual substances themselves. After my first set of blood results, he kept my thyroid medication at the same dose and prescribed Metformin, a medication given for Type 2 diabetics. Even though my glucose levels appeared fine, he hoped my body responded better to insulin. The drug would decrease the amount of sugar made by the liver and inhibit its absorption into my body. This was a concept I clearly understood. I believed Metformin could provide the results I wanted, if I actually fell into this category of Insulin Resistance.

I had walked into the appointment aware that this particular endocrinologist followed conventional methods for treating his patients. I wasn't exactly ecstatic that he downplayed Functional Medicine, but I found myself relieved to have a hiatus from my current protocol. I had given that regimen more than ample time to work its magic and I was more than ready to give prescriptive medication another chance, costing me $450 at every appointment.

By late fall of 2010, I lost a few more pounds after raising my Metformin dosage from 500 to 2000 milligrams, taking four pills a day. I continued avoiding gluten, soy, dairy and peanuts, and exercised with moderation, using a trainer twice a week, thirty minutes each time. My medical appointments were spread out monthly and finally played a secondary role in my life. As the numbers on the scale decreased, I found more options in my wardrobe, leaving me with a sense of peace. I believed I was slowly but surely approaching the finish line.

A couple months later, I came home from the movies in the evening to find a note on the kitchen counter. It was a phone number of a missed call from one of my sister's friends, whose third child was in my daughters' class. A half hour later we were on the phone, discussing her husband's health condition which had plummeted over the last seven months. The more details she provided, the more it seemed Adam had giardia, and I insisted on speaking with him.

Was it possible I found someone else in the same predicament who actually lived in my neighborhood? Despite our proximity, we only met a few times over the years. I had little memory of Adam's build, other than being average height and sporting a buzz cut. It was hard to imagine him with the same bloated belly as me.

When Adam got on the phone, complaining of exhaustion, discomfort in his abdomen and extreme bloat among other issues, he immediately brought me back to those miserable days. I wondered if his bloat was a bit exaggerated, assuming only a woman could look the way I did, with the same basketball-shaped belly. I sympathized with his every complaint and offered any worthwhile advice I received from certain doctors—something I had wished for during my recovery. After Adam shared his struggles with

Colitis, mentioning he already had a point person leading his case, I stood silent, questioning which referral suited him.

I suggested Dr. Cahill, knowing he was the only doctor whose giardia test was valid.

"Make an appointment with him, since all you need is a confirmation."

This was our first real conversation, but I sensed it wouldn't be our last if I could offer more guidance. "You have to let me know when you hear something. It's got to be a match!"

A week later, Adam called, confirming he tested positive for giardia. It took two rounds of antibiotics before he would test negative. Once he was clear, I sent him to my latest endocrinologist, helping him avoid the unnecessary expenses Jeff and I had incurred. Over the next few months, Adam and I checked in with each other on a regular basis, comparing protocols. At times we even laughed, acknowledging the various doctors we had seen and our collective aggravation over the lack of answers. I appreciated Adam's candor and ability to repeat the doctor's clarifications verbatim after his appointments, something I couldn't do. After all this time feeling so alone with my condition, I had finally found camaraderie with a neighbor.

On the days Adam had setbacks, we commiserated together, amazed how another human being truly understood the depths of this illness. We didn't have to imagine how each other felt—we actually experienced it. Even though we suffered from most of the same symptoms, some impacted us differently. When the fatigue was at its worst and left me lethargic, I slept the days away. Adam didn't have that luxury because he was running his company to support his family; he couldn't afford to allow the exhaustion of the illness to affect his business: distributing shipping supplies while processing volumes of paperwork and driving to see clients on a daily basis.

By comparison, I didn't have much to complain about and could not fathom doing what he did. When I shared my frustrations about weight gain, Adam, not surprisingly, was unsympathetic. "That's the least of my concerns," he said.

I wished weight gain had been the least of my worries, but my body image continued to haunt me whenever I looked in the mirror and remembered my former self. I was trapped in the evil vortex of comparison, and couldn't get past the issue no matter what the giardia was trying to teach me.

"Keep me posted. You're going to get through this," I said to Adam, but really meant to remind myself—even though I was feeling better. I trusted Adam would get there one day, too.

CHAPTER
19

B Y MAY 2011, my energy had returned in full force, even after I stopped taking vitamin B12 injections. Now conscious of the intensity I inflicted on my body, the compulsion to over-exert myself during workouts vanished. It was time I found a healthy balance of activity, so I could show some self-restraint on the days my figure seemed flawed. I was able to maintain a moderate exercise regimen and appreciated the morning runs that I once believed were long gone. I had the pleasure of Buddy's company on a daily basis and could finally bask in his affection and presence.

One morning, Buddy watched as I dressed in gym clothes and waited patiently by the garage door while I dropped the girls at school. Upon my return, his tail wagged with excitement, knowing he was seconds from enjoying some fresh air. Most times, he kept up with my pace, eyes focused on the road as he trotted through the neighborhood.

On occasion, when Buddy got distracted by another dog, car or squirrel, I tugged his leash, making sure he followed my lead. Every time we approached the last hill, one hundred feet from home, I looked at Buddy and declared, "Ready Boo? First one to the garage door wins." Then I dropped his leash, sprinting as fast as possible, hoping one day I'd outrun him.

I made sure his bowls of food and water were filled before I headed towards my bedroom. While I showered, Buddy kept me company and lay on my bathroom floor. When I initiated conversation, he raised those heavy eyebrows in response, enjoying his newfound attention. The days of neglect were history. As I left the bathroom, he changed positions and rested on the decorative wool pillows which he recently claimed as his own.

One evening at Buddy's bedtime, he charmed us into sleeping in our room as opposed to his crate. I chuckled as I watched Jeff play a twenty minute game of tag around our bed until Buddy stopped on the side of my bed where I rested. He tilted his head in my direction, with those desperate droopy eyes begging for my approval, as if my sickness had never occurred. I petted his head.

"Aw Jeff, look at him. I think it's time to dump the crate," I said, knowing Buddy was two years old.

Jeff agreed. Buddy licked my fingers in excitement but I yanked my hand away.

"Ugh, just no licking, okay," I said, pointing my index finger at his snout. I immediately ran to the bathroom and washed my hands because his saliva was still a sore spot for me.

When Jeff and I were settled in bed, Buddy plopped down on my side and slept through the night. The next morning, we found him on the floor at the foot of our bed asleep on his side, head propped on a wool pillow, like a human. He looked as peaceful as I now felt, and he gave those pillows a permanent place on our bedroom floor. Sometimes now we find him curled

up there with a blanket wrapped around him, obviously provided
by the girls.

In May, my parents insisted on a fortieth birthday luncheon to celebrate the new me. I was eager to oblige, appreciating my good health.
Giardia had given me a second take on life; now I could look beyond
just my body image, as opposed to how I spent my last two birthdays.

For the first time in three years, phone conversations with my
mother didn't revolve around dreadful updates about my health.
Even when my father answered, he didn't pass the phone off.
Instead, I shared with him the appreciation I had for my children,
including Buddy's recent mishaps, when I found the girls'
'blind' dolls whose eyes he had chewed off. Lately, Buddy
seemed to be a magician and Jeff was his assistant. Instead of pulling handkerchiefs from a clown's mouth, Jeff delicately removed
the rest of a thinly-roped dog toy from Buddy's rear end, which
resulted in laughter from our entire family.

I continued to meet friends and spend time with family, enjoying the benefits of my good health. Every improvement reinforced
my conscientious food plan. At this point, I gained an enormous
amount of nutritional knowledge. Between the dozen or more
medical protocols and plethora of professional advice, I could
discern which foods worked best for my body.

I still avoided gluten, soy, dairy and peanuts because they
appeared on every allergen test. I reintroduced egg whites after
no bloating resulted, wondering if afternoon cleanses contributed to this harmony. My meals were consistent. I ate egg whites
with an orange for breakfast. For lunch, I ate a salad with chick-
en, a healthy fat—avocado, sliced almonds or walnuts—a small
portion of a fresh mango or apple, and used olive or flaxseed oil
as dressings. In the late afternoon, I made a shake consisting of

water, any berry, and the same cleansing powder that was once suggested to me by the same 'mad scientist' with the hocus pocus oils. Dinner afforded me the most variety and choices: grilled turkey burger, shrimp, chicken or salmon. I combined the protein with either steamed or sautéed vegetables, added garlic, olive oil and lemon and ate that with quinoa, millet or brown rice. On occasion, I skipped the grain and savored my favorite vegetable instead, roasted butternut squash. Dessert was always an apple.

My friends wondered when I would add other foods back into my diet, but I insisted on my new regimen because I looked as good as I felt. All this time, no one had judged my choices. My friends showed genuine concern for me with their questions about the different protocols, food allergies or Ziploc bags crammed with supplements.

When it was time for me to try certain foods again, they followed my announcements with enthusiastic applause.

"I'm eating whole-wheat pasta, edamame and frozen yogurt again without bloating!"

Now that I felt better and had more food options, my meals no longer resembled science projects to others. The perplexed looks had vanished from most of my friends' faces and left me at ease while we ate. I even reclaimed ownership of my handbag, leaving the many Ziploc bags of supplements at home. I cleared the kitchen counter top by sweeping my arm across the three feet of half-used supplement bottles into a large shopping bag, then stored it in the back of the laundry room closet. My life seemed normal again.

While I wasn't the original size two from my marathon days, I felt a sense of contentment for the very first time in ages. Though I wasn't deriving love from my self-image alone, I would be lying if I didn't acknowledge the thrill I got every time I opened my closet doors, pleased to see the large selection of clothes I could finally wear. No matter what pair of jeans I grabbed, they fit, sliding over my thighs without applied force, sweat or tears.

The full-length mirror that once had humbled me, now projected a more graceful, content woman. My skin glowed, a sign that my body was absorbing all its nutrients; however, I still worried about the hair test. I was terrified I'd wake up one day with bald spots after repeatedly finding clumps of hair woven between my fingers every morning over the last couple of years, which I tossed into the bathroom garbage. But that morning, when I raised my hand towards my head, spreading each finger to gently rake through a section of my hair, I felt the thickness and texture that had been missing for months. My heart pounded and I slowly opened my eyes and looked down at my hand, without finding a single strand of hair. The thyroid medication was finally at its correct dosage.

The tinkling of Buddy's collar interrupted me. I saw him in the mirror, devouring his leg, like a Thanksgiving feast. I assumed his incessant licking was partly due to boredom since he just finished breakfast and was waiting for me to stop preening and leave the room.

I whistled. "No licking."

Buddy raised his head, staring at my reflection in the mirror. I squinted, noticing the quarter-sized pink irritation in place of his fur and knelt to get a closer look. His paw was raw and needed attention. I immediately called the veterinarian for an appointment, trying to squeeze it in between visits to the hospital to see my mother-in-law, Ilene, who had suffered a heart attack a few weeks back, which had sent shockwaves through our family.

I took Buddy to the vet during one of my breaks from the hospital, where I had volunteered myself to be Ilene's advocate, empathizing with all the sadness and frustration she felt after losing all control over her everyday affairs. Though it was not my intention, most hours of my day were dedicated to looking after Ilene in the hospital. I was playing another disappearing act on my daughters, but I could not ignore the medical attention Buddy needed. The veterinarian assumed his sore resulted from excessive licking, possibly due to food allergies. I chuckled at the coincidence while he reiterated the commonality among dogs.

"There's a test to confirm his allergies but it costs $500 or you can just change his food and see if he gets better."

My eyes widened. I instantly agreed to the latter after imagining the look on Jeff's face and hearing how much I spent on our dog's allergen test.

"Can I get his new food at a pet store?" I asked, noticing the slight quiver of my leg. How much extra would that cost us? I would rather have been at Ilene's bedside than try to figure out this problem. Holding her hand was a lot easier than holding Buddy's health together.

"Absolutely," he said, suggesting we switch to Natural Balance, salmon and sweet potato flavor. I felt my chest tighten again, aware I was holding my breath. The vet walked me to the reception area and gave me a prescription for steroids, hoping to relieve the itchiness and swelling from Buddy's inflammation, a term I now understood and heard often. I checked the prescription label, struck by the similarities in our medications. How unfortunate that the treatments weren't timed better. I would have suggested to Jeff that I take Buddy's meds instead of my own when I was prescribed antibiotics—and save us a boatload in prescription expenses.

"The licking should stop in the next few days," the vet said.

On my way back to my mother-in-law's hospital room, I shared the latest news with Jeff. I hoped he would see the humor but he only focused on the cost of the test, despite the fact that I reiterated we weren't going to run it. I sat down on the tip of Ilene's bed, sharing the results of Buddy's appointment with her. Within moments, I noticed a familiar face standing next to the nurse's station through the sliding glass doors. I jumped off the edge of her bed and headed in his direction.

"Dr. Zacharias," I shouted, revealing a huge grin.

He looked up from his file and smiled. "Berko!" He gave me a huge hug.

"It's been a while. What are you doing here?"

I pointed towards Ilene's room, briefly explaining her situation which, while not ideal, was improving every day. I was bursting to tell him the other good news. "This is the real me!"

He stood quiet, confused by my comment.

I spread my fingers wide and grabbed my waist. "This is what I actually look like!"

He stared at me a moment and smiled, then reached out and put his hand on my shoulder.

"It's good to see you healthy."

I shared a condensed version of my eighteen-month journey to health, broaching the different protocols from boiling the backyard dirt and the search for a simple strainer. He continuously shook his head in amazement. "Sounds pretty simple to me," he said, giving me the same comforting wink. "I hope I don't see you anytime soon."

"You won't," I promised and flashed him one last smile on my way back to Ilene's room.

The good news continued through the end of June. I met with my endocrinologist for a six month follow-up appointment to learn about my latest test results. He looked up from his file with relief. "Your numbers look perfect," he said and handed me prescriptions for the next six months of refills. Perfect? The word sounded so good I had to pause and savor it. I was relieved that my regimen had been reduced to only two medications, Armour Thyroid and Metformin, and one daily probiotic, which I would take regardless of any health issue. On the way out of his office, I made my final payment of $450 from our giardia fund.

When the girls left for their second summer at camp, I wrote letters daily and even stamped dog paws onto Buddy's own stationary after Jolie insisted she get "more letters in the mail from Buddy."

I even sent the girls an email before Buddy and I began our days with an early run around the neighborhood. One morning, I kept the sliding door open in the kitchen, shutting only the screen. Buddy sunned himself on the deck while I took a shower and blasted the iPod. When I turned off the water, I was startled to see him in the bathroom.

I opened the shower door and grabbed a towel, quickly drying off my body. Buddy sat motionless with a mischievous look on his face, waiting for a reaction. I wrapped the towel around my middle, deducing the ways in which he got there. "Who's so smart," I said, convinced he opened the screen door himself. Then it occurred to me that he might have broken the screen door. I feared the worst from Jeff. He was incredibly stressed from work and trying to repair the damage of my past medical costs that even replacing a screen on our sliding door would cause aggravation. He didn't need to be burdened with additional mishaps.

"Oh my god!" I screeched.

I wrapped the towel tightly around my body and ran toward the kitchen as Buddy trailed behind. I stopped, catching a glimpse of the screen door—wide open. I glanced down at Buddy, who waited patiently for my affection. I dropped to my knees and hugged him tightly. "Wait until the girls learn about this," I said, eager to write the next batch of camp letters.

CHAPTER
20

B Y OCTOBER 2011, I was committed to understanding the big
picture about giardia. I was also very concerned about the others
who still struggled with this condition. Despite most doctors' fears, I
turned to the Internet, learning everything I could about the parasite. I had not surfed the web for fourteen months, assuming my doctors had all the information; however, I needed to trust my intuition
now since I had already correctly diagnosed myself from the outset.

I spent thirty hours per week in front of the computer immersed
in research while Buddy took countless naps at the foot of my bedside. When he woke up, he nuzzled his nose against my laptop.
Aside from taking care of the girls, I became obsessed with learning
every intricate detail written about giardia.

When I stumbled upon the www.medicine.net statistics, I sat in
silence, floored by the number of people walking around with this

infection. Most people I knew had never heard of giardia. When I searched for the words "carrier", "giardiasis" and "United States" together, I found a result on diet.com. I clicked the link even though this particular site seemed unrelated to my topic. I skimmed the article and learned that 15% of people who swallow giardia cysts are asymptomatic. The cases are usually detected only if the person's stool is tested during a community outbreak, hence my husband's testing positive. This was an important concept to grasp, but too often missed: people with cysts in their digestive tracts can still transmit giardia even if they don't develop any symptoms.

People with cysts in their digestive tracts can still transmit giardia regardless of developing any symptoms.

I reread that statement several times, comprehending the magnitude of undiagnosed cases. Without my diagnosis, Jeff would have never learned he was infected. Could he have had it as long as I did, being asymptomatic the whole time? Or was I the source of his transmission at some point during my condition? My germaphobe mind reeled when I considered how many times Jeff had prepared the girls' meals. If this was true for my family, then millions of Americans were living with chronic conditions like I had, or worse, were carriers like Jeff, continuously spreading this infection unbeknownst to them. I was hungry for more evidence.

Most staggering, I learned that approximately 80% of water samples from lakes, streams and ponds in the United States contained giardia, according to CDC reports.

While I was aware that cysts lived in cool and wet conditions for several months, the veterinarian never gave me any percentages on infection rates for humans and animals. Horrified, I thought about Hurricane Irene's aftermath at the end of August 2011, which was the seventh costliest hurricane in the history of the United States. According to Wikipedia, the widespread damage was estimated at $15.6 billion dollars and caused over 56 deaths. Extreme flooding occurred all along the East Coast due to overflowing rivers and lakes. At that time, I was as diligent as anyone when it came to storm preparation, accumulating the basic necessities if we lost electricity. I even refused to drink the tap water from restaurants, wondering if they coånsistently boiled their water to eliminate germs. But it never occurred to me that the water had not been tested specifically for giardia after the hurricane.

I looked up the CDC to find any data that related to contaminated drinking water but couldn't find any statistics documented after the storm. The most recent information reported was listed under the giardiasis surveillance, 2009–2010, which stated the risks of using untreated groundwater from either poorly built or damaged wells. Most frequent diagnosis reporting occurred in northern states, implicating drinking water as an important vehicle for transmitting giardia. I wondered how many people had been drinking this kind of water before receiving any precautions about boiling it first? I imagined the streams that ran through so many of the properties near our home. My heart sank when I thought about Buddy and other dogs drinking contaminated water. Of all the findings I had discovered, none struck me more than this. No one reported that these areas were contaminated during the hurricane—that indeed, untreated water in our own backyards carried giardia and could make us incredibly sick.

The CDC concluded that the burden and cost of acute giardiasis in the United States cost nearly $34 million in hospitalizations. I had spent more than $50,000 just to recover from my condition alone, and I represented 1 of 2.5 million Americans. I wondered why, if this report was made public, hospitals didn't test for giardia, considering it would cut the cost of treatment significantly? During all my emergency room visits, I was told hospitals only dealt with the acute problem at hand, which only related to my stool. If I had been tested immediately, I could have received answers and antibiotics within twenty-four hours.

I continued my research and found topix.com, a site devoted to a community of giardia sufferers who shared their stories and treatments. I read over a thousand posts from all over the world dating back to 2006. Everyone seemed to be in my same situation, grasping at straws while trying to get cured. Even more disheartening was realizing there was still no consistent evidence of a recovery. I was more amazed to see the number of people who relapsed on and off over a period of years, grateful for my comparatively short three year journey and the fact I was clean.

The most distressing discovery was that giardia had been consistently misdiagnosed as chronic fatigue, irritable bowel syndrome and depression. My journey had been lived by many: children, who had the highest rates of infection; and adults, mostly women aged 30–45. Contamination happened through contact with daycare centers, water parks and household pets, and by traveling to foreign countries..

I wondered why the test wasn't mandatory for all puppies? A handful of my friends had asked their veterinarian to test their own puppy in light of my experience. A few had tested positive for giardia. At least my friends were now aware of transmission.

I needed an expert to help me sift through and validate my research. The only person I trusted was Dr. Galland, who had written many articles and had studied this issue at great length— and had also suffered from giardia himself.

At the end of October, we spent some time on the phone. He listed ways the infection was transferred and made distinctions between the two types of symptoms: people suffering from an acute problem versus chronic problem. He recited each symptom then clarified why some people could experience other unusual symptoms—suggesting the connection to one's immune response—which can be triggered by giardia. I was taken aback as he ran through some of the unusual symptoms: joint pain, an overgrowth of bacteria and yeast in the small intestine, neurological effects such as brain fog, and waves of fatigue after meals. He had confirmed my chronic case, and solved the mystery of why some doctors questioned if I had Hypoglycemia or Insulin Resistance. Finally, the facts were beginning to make sense.

Dr. Galland explained how a person is more susceptible to acquiring giardia based on the condition of their immune system. Once again, I knew my past behavior had contributed significantly to making my body prone to complications caused by giardia. By not paying attention to my body over the years—and focusing only on my image and the numbers on a scale—I had overlooked what my body needed to stay strong and resist the power of a parasite.

Dr. Galland cited information from a study done on animals whose intestines weren't damaged by giardia even after certain aspects of their immune system were disabled.

"The immune system produces the damage of giardia, resulting in hives and arthritis," he said.

Memories of running in the rain while on antibiotics for a double infection flashed through my head like a reproach.

Still, I questioned why weight gain played a major role in my condition, especially since so many websites cited weight loss as a top symptom. He went into further detail, describing the immune system as a complex set of reactions compromised by stress. This was the first time I heard stress was related to giardia.

"When you get sick with something else, the way your body responds to the other illness might actually activate giardia," he said, recalling numerous timeswhen I needed antibiotics for my sinus infections, strep throat and pink eye. He further described this double-edge sword. Any immune suppression through high doses of steroids or otherwise, interferes with the ability to clear giardia. Immune activation contributes to the inflammation associated with the infection, explaining why my colds or flu only got worse. After taking a high dose of Cortef for four months, I wondered if my grossly distended abdomen had any relation to my hormonal imbalances.

Based on the lack of studies, it was uncertain if giardia harms a person's hormones more than other types of chronic infections. I was reminded of the conversations with my acupuncturist about what triggered an autoimmune response. He gave an example of a patient who first showed signs of Lupus at age fifty, only after experiencing a chronic infection.

Dr. Galland distinguished between the two different tests that confirm diagnoses. The stool test was the standard and most common test done by hospital labs and national diagnostic labs. All my stool tests missed giardia.

According to Dr. Galland, a single stool test will only pick up 50% of cases and multiple stool tests are still inaccurate 10% of the time, even in acute giardiasis. The second stool test is the rectal swab test and isn't used by most physicians or tropical medicine specialists. However, Dr. Cahill and a few other parasitologists use this test to confirm a diagnosis, including mine. Since the infection is located in the small intestine, this test can often find giardia cysts. Although invasive, this swab test takes only ten minutes and could be the easiest and most direct solution for hospitals. I was shocked to hear this because it was never mentioned on the Internet or suggested in a report.

Dr. Galland reviewed treatments and their side effects, and ran through the various options, beginning with the oldest antibiotics available to the newest on the market. The last topic he covered was diet, since nutrition significantly impacted one's symptoms.

"It may take months, a year or even longer before you are able to eat a normal diet after having giardia." He suggested eliminating foods that aggravate one's symptoms, noting sensitivity to sugar found in fruits, sweets, alcohol and wheat, and offered a few different diets. This is why I was recommended nutritional supplements: to offset deficiency in Vitamins A and B12. He advised those who appeared to be cured but still had symptoms to get tested for Small Intestinal Bacterial Overgrowth. The Internet was extremely vague regarding food sensitivities after a patient healed, and it did not provide any helpful diets.

By the end of the summer, I was well aware that I had gained back some weight, but I hadn't experienced any bloat this time and wasn't overly concerned. I wondered what constituted the bloat and fatigue since those symptoms were once at the top of my list of complaints.

I believed there was an absolute connection with taking hormones and my pregnant-sized belly even though no evidence existed. How bloated did I need to be to prove my theory? It had been two years since I was infected, but I wondered if I had waited long enough for my digestive tract to recover, or if I would have to avoid sensitive foods forever.

One evening that fall, I bumped into Adam and his sixteen year -old son while they were eating frozen yogurt. Our correspondence had ended over the summer because our conditions had become manageable; however, we immediately updated each other on our health. I forced a smile, downplaying the recent weight gain and beginning signs of sluggish energy. Adam mentioned his distended abdomen and the fatigue that had returned, and I pointed to my stomach, revealing my own thickening waistline, sharing his frustration. His son stared at us perplexed, then made the association and said, "Oh right, the parasite lady."

I forced a smile. "Yeah, right," I said, hoping no one else remembered me that way.

On the ride home, I worried about Dr. Galland's assessments about my diet after hearing that Adam's symptoms had returned. It was time to accept that the foods I had added back over the summer were causing my latest symptoms. I could no longer afford to play the victim, feeling as if I was being 'denied' any lasting eating pleasures. I was alive and I needed to start focusing on my wellbeing, not the foods I could no longer eat. If I didn't have my health, nothing would bring me lasting pleasure.

By winter, I found another way to distract myself from my goal of being healthy. I pulled all nighters working on this book, but my body was not responding like a college student. Instead of staring at my belly in the full-length mirror, I fixated on the exhaustion on my face.

One morning after a late night writing spree, I woke up half alert, stepping in a pile of Buddy's vomit. "What the hell?" I growled, rubbing my eyes, insisting that Jeff race out of bed to get paper towels. I waited, balancing on one leg, with the dirty foot dangling in midair.

Jeff turned on the lights, revealing two other piles. He approached the foot of the bed and kneeled down beside Buddy, sprawled on his decorative wool pillows.

"Boo, you feeling alright?"

I stared at my foot, sickened by the thought of microscopic creatures crawling around this horrid mess. "Uh, hello? I'm the one with the dog's vomit on my foot," I said, motioning for attention.

Jeff chuckled, "Hey Buddy, I think mommy's upset you gave her the cooties."

He ripped off a few sheets of paper towel from the roll and wiped my foot. I went to the bathroom and sat on the toilet, grabbing fistfuls of disinfecting wipes to scrub my foot, praying to avoid another infection.

Jeff cleaned off Buddy's paws while the girls ate breakfast. I could hear Jolie giggling.

"You have to show us again. What did mom's face look like?" she asked.

"I'm so glad my germaphobic moments entertain all of you," I said, walking in on their conversation while describing the possible critters that could have been crawling on my foot.

Abby got up from the table and headed towards the garbage, rolling her eyes. "Great, Mom, now you're going to make your kids nuts, too."

It certainly wasn't my intention to create phobias, but after the research I'd done over the last few months, I couldn't avoid it. I worried incessantly about Buddy's licks. I worried about the girls forgetting to wash their hands before meals, if they drank from public water fountains or any unfiltered water, or touched restroom door handles. Who handled their food in restaurants? Did my girls keep their mouths shut as they swam in the lake at camp? Was someone responsible for informing my daughters about potential outbreaks? Could I get them to be so grossed out by porta potties that they'd avoid using them altogether? Yes, I wanted control. I wanted us to live a life where none of these questions mattered. But they did matter and I could not let go.

"Seriously mom, please stop!" Jolie and Abby said, as if they could read my mind.

I took my new mission seriously. If no one was appointed to tell the public about giardia, or help others who suffered from it, I would. I enrolled in a 10-week leadership course that fall, building my confidence in public speaking so I could raise awareness.

One night during the drive, Jeff called, frazzled.

"Buddy's got a huge gash in his leg and I can't stop the bleeding."

My stomach dropped as I gripped the steering wheel. I had left him outside, roaming our backyard for two hours while I waited for Jeff to come home from work. During one of Buddy's late afternoon bathroom breaks, I found dark brown streaks on the fur on his neck, back and ears. I grabbed a towel when Buddy came in the kitchen and prepared to clean him off until I got close enough and took a whiff, smelling a foul odor: somehow he had managed to roll in his own feces. I immediately backed away, repulsed by the thought of touching him. I sent him back outside until Jeff could hose him down. My family knew I banned myself from any contact with Buddy's stool, unless he relieved himself during one of our morning runs. In those cases, I whipped out my rubber gloves and double bagged his poo.

"Oh my God! Did he get that while I left him outside?" I asked, feeling horribly guilty.

"Forget about that for a minute. I'm worried he needs stitches," Jeff said.

Stitches? My eyes widened as he continued, "There was blood everywhere in the shower and the girls are freaking out."

I overheard crying in the background and felt a large pit in my stomach.

"Who's crying?"

Jeff sighed, "Abby, she saw part of his bone."

"Bone? Wait, how big is the gash?" I asked, insisting Jeff take Buddy to the animal hospital since our veterinarian's office was closed. I glanced at the highway signs, deciding if I should get off the nearest exit and head home.

"The hole's a decent size," he said, "Just do me a favor, call the animal hospital first since it's twenty minutes from the house and ask if it's necessary. Maybe we can wrap it and wait until the vet's office hours tomorrow."

We were told he needed immediate attention and both of us knew the expense would be doubled. Buddy returned with seven stitches and a cast. I was on the phone with my mother when he pushed open our bedroom door wearing a lampshade-sized cone tied around his neck.

I hung up and walked over to him, touching the sides of his face, feeling full of remorse. His eyes looked groggy from the anesthesia. He limped toward his pillows at the end of our bed and I helped him lay down, positioning his cone in a way that was comfortable. I rested beside him, face-to-face, feeling every pang of guilt while he cried on and off through the night.

CHAPTER
21

B Y FEBRUARY 2012, I was finally ready to face my new reality —exhausted, slightly bloated and carrying extra weight. I grabbed a few dresses from our basement cedar closet and tried them on for my nephew's upcoming Bar Mitzvah in March. My body barely squeezed into any of the dresses regardless of their style, and I noticed the materials pulled tightly around my hips, midsection and thighs.

Once again, I found myself standing in front of the mirror, glaring at my weight gain. Twelve pounds on a woman twice my size would not be a big deal, but it didn't leave much room for hiding anything on my petite frame. I was speechless as the tears slid down my cheeks. Dark puffy circles hung beneath my eyes and I regretted the many sleepless nights throughout this ordeal, but for the first time, I realized there was no one to blame but myself.

I had lived my whole life inside this distorted perception of who I was based on my appearance. Was *this* the point of the giardia? Was *this* the message hidden inside all those microorganisms? Was I finally waking up to their message: you are not what you look like. You are not what you think. I was a stranger to myself then, but I knew I needed medical attention, again.

I scheduled an appointment with my endocrinologist, bracing for the $450 expense we'd incur and the conversation I'd have with Jeff. I canceled at the last minute, unable to bear any more conflict in our family, but something else stopped me: if I returned to the same treatment, I'd get the same results. It was simple. I needed an alternative approach to taking Armour Thyroid and Metformin, which caused more weight gain despite my strict diet. I needed a fresh perspective from a doctor who practiced Functional Medicine with experience in women's hormones and metabolisms.

My sister-in-law, Marcy, recommended I see her doctor who had an extensive background in anti-aging programs, bio-identical hormones and metabolic makeovers, which covered a person's physical and mental state through nutritional and supplemental care. It is known that a woman's metabolism slows down once they reach their forties. I wasn't a spring chicken anymore and needed to recognize that weight loss wasn't as easy as it was in the past. Marcy recently lost more than twenty pounds by following one of the doctor's regimens. It was worth a shot.

I appreciated the amount of time this doctor gave me over the phone, observing her calming disposition. I scanned her website for further validation. It seemed a perfect fit after reading her accomplishments and willingness to bring vibrancy back to her patients' lives.

A week later, I sat in her office with my medical records dating back to August 2010. The doctor was in her late forties. She was slender, had short brown hair and not a wrinkle on her face, which I hoped was proof her treatments worked well. I kept my history brief since we had already spoken on the phone.

"I won't take hormones after the terrible reactions I experienced," I said, using my hands to mime the basketball-shaped belly I once had. She listened intently as I described the list of food allergies that occurred over the last four years. I also addressed my current level of exhaustion. "I'm done taking Metformin and am willing to try anything to lose this additional weight," I said, leaning forward and sorting through my endocrinologist's blood tests. I pulled the latest results from June and the first metabolic workup I had done ten months prior.

I waited for answers while she reviewed the paperwork.

"Sometimes blood doesn't prove a patient's symptoms very well," she said, and then asked me about the severity of my bloat, irritability, weakness and fatigue. She refused to prescribe anything until she ran a complete blood workup, covering my metabolic breakdown, and suggested I avoid using hormones.

"It seems your reaction was caused by the parasite and you shouldn't have any further complications since it's been eradicated for over two years."

I was confident that my bout with giardia was long gone.

The doctor put my mind at ease by acknowledging other weight loss options, namely the HCG diet, knowing it provided many of her patients with quick results. Human Chronic Gonadotripin is a hormone the body produces and is most commonly associated with women's pregnancies. It was first discovered in 1927 but it wasn't until the 1950s when a doctor figured out that HCG also suppressed appetites and stimulated weight loss and muscle development. I had heard about HCG from my sister-in-law and from a Dr. Oz episode, but the side effects of taking a synthetic version gave me pause. The doctor offered a logical explanation, relieving my fears. It seemed this low calorie diet didn't make the body experience deprivation, and instead tricked it into believing it was getting thousands of calories a day.

By combining HCG and a five-hundred calorie diet, the body believes it needs to use the stored fat for energy and removes the excess fat reserves. Apparently, this natural process has no negative effects on one's metabolism and results in weight loss of between a half a pound and three pounds daily.

She explained that in resetting the hypothalamus and pituitary gland, it then encourages the endocrine system and hormones to reset. The metabolism reacts differently and people have an easier time maintaining future weight loss. At this point, I wasn't about to waste another year of my life on medications, supplements and a variety of regimens. All I knew was that my hypothalamus controlled the communication to my thyroid, adrenal glands, metabolism and other hormones. I figured this was the perfect way to reset my system, erasing the memory of giardia for good. The treatment had fast and reliable results, which left me easily convinced. As long as I had sufficient sleeping habits and beginning signs of weight loss, I'd feel great again in no time.

The doctor offered the medication in one of two ways: placing liquid droplets underneath the tongue or by giving subcutaneous injections into the abdomen. I chose the latter, claiming expertise at giving myself shots. Before starting, she wanted me to take a saliva test to confirm that my cortisol levels were in decent shape. "It takes three weeks to receive results," she said.

I didn't want to go through that test again even though I was told numerous times that saliva was more reliable than blood work. I figured my cortisol levels were fine, so what would be the point in prolonging the weight loss? "Can't I skip the test?" I asked, reminding her that I knew the difference between my levels of fatigue. "I'd rather not wait another month."

The doctor straightened. "Are you sure?" she asked. "I don't think that's a great idea."

I pushed harder. "If my blood work shows I'm eligible, then I'll be fine," I said, reiterating the many rigid food plans I already followed.

She was silent for a moment. "As long as everything looks good on your blood test." She wrote up a tentative protocol and handed me a stack of papers, explaining the details of the diet. Phase one lasted twenty-six days and consisted of a small list of selected foods: one tablespoon of milk at breakfast, one fruit eaten as a mid morning snack, three and a half ounces of protein combined with a cup of vegetables for lunch, a second fruit eaten as a mid afternoon snack, and dinner was chosen from the same list of lunch foods without repeating meals. I was allowed tea, coffee and water throughout the day and the use of only one lemon, besides other basic seasonings—but I already avoided dairy, tea and coffee, further limiting my options.

We had scheduled a few office visits during phase one and planned on corresponding via email. I left her office with optimism and a list of nutritional supplements needed to shift my body's imbalances, including DHEA, fish oil and a multivitamin.

I pushed for everything. I wanted those shots and would have said anything for the doctor's permission. In the end, she gave in because the blood work showed my cortisol levels were fine. I was caught in an unbreakable web of panic, and I refused to gain any more weight.

I expected a phone call from the doctor during the girls' February break, but heard from Adam first. "I'm on my second round of antibiotics. I can't get rid of this freaking parasite," he said, keeping the details brief because he was on vacation with his family.

I listened, shocked, sensing his frustration. I wanted to help him by sharing more of what I had learned, but didn't want to overwhelm him, recalling the countless suggestions I had already made. He had been cleared of giardia for almost seven months—and now he was saying it was back. How was this even possible? I hung up, feeling gripped by sudden despair. The last thing I wanted to consider was that my recent weight gain had anything to do with giardia.

I focused on the latest diet. It wasn't as easy as I thought. I ate the allotted amount of calories per day, but my fatigue worsened. Instead of stopping to reflect on what was happening, I pushed harder and harder. This diet was going to work come hell or high water because there was no way I was willing to acknowledge the alternative. I could not have giardia again.

I checked in with the doctor through email. Worried that I wasn't getting enough energy, she suggested I increase my daily calories, insisting I add more protein and suggesting other supplements to boost my energy levels. I hesitated, welcoming only a diet that would slim my waistline. A few days before my nephew's Bar Mitzvah, I made another appointment.

I sat in the doctor's office while she expressed concern over my headaches and increased exhaustion. "I think it's time to stop the diet altogether. I'm really worried about you. The fatigue and headaches should have lifted by now."

"The weekend is coming up and I'll make sure to rest. I want to keep doing this. If I feel worse, then I'll stop," I said, like an addict bullying my dealer. Relaxation wasn't in the cards for me that weekend, and I refused to relent on the diet. I was so wrapped up in my old behaviors that I ignored every warning sign my body provided.

After the Bar Mitzvah, my family drove home from Westchester, New York. I stared at the highway, wondering if the three extra pounds I had "lost" that morning had been worth the effort. Though I was relieved to have lost eleven pounds by then, I couldn't deny the shakiness from the fatigue any longer. I felt like hell. Between the car rides, evening and morning temple services, and the reception, my body had hit a wall.

I caught Jeff looking at me and hid my trembling fingers inside my thighs. He touched my shoulder and asked, "What's the matter? You feel alright?"

I gently pulled away and refused eye contact, embarrassed to tell him the truth. "Just tired from the weekend. As soon as we get home, I'm getting into bed," I said.

I dragged myself out of bed the next morning at 9:30. My legs felt like cement bricks as I lifted them, one at a time, onto the scale. I waited until the blue number was clear and read 119 lbs. I stood stunned, realizing I gained three pounds overnight without deviating from the diet. My head pounded and my body felt weak. I slowly made my way to the kitchen, grabbed my cell phone off the counter and headed back to bed, stepping over Buddy's sleeping body. I emailed the doctor, expressing serious concerns, and labeled the message urgent.

I took my mother's suggestion and stayed in bed for the rest of the day. I was grateful for Buddy's company while he rested at the foot of my bed. Anxious, I kept checking my phone for the doctor's response. *Meet me in my office tomorrow at 10 a.m.*

I found a substitute to fill in for me at school the next day and called the head teacher.

The following morning, I could barely brush my hair and pull it into a ponytail. I put on gym pants and a sweatshirt and slogged

my way to the doctor, and sat lifeless in her office. I never imagined a day when I'd feel this low again.

"I can see the difference in your energy just by looking at
you," the doctor said.

"I don't even feel like I'm in my body anymore," I said, regretting that I skipped the saliva test, which evaluated the levels of my
cortisol before I started the diet. "Now what?"

She insisted on more blood tests. "Clearly, your adrenal
glands weren't in the shape you thought," she said, suspecting
it suppressed my immune system and strained my hormones.
"In the meantime, take the saliva test. It's possible you'll need
additional hormone support to help raise those levels. Let's see
what shows up on your blood work."

I struggled to make eye contact with her, incredulous that I
was back in this predicament, worrying about my cortisol levels.
She knew my reservations about taking hormones and I trusted
her, knowing this was her area of expertise. She was the first doctor
I met who was trained in bio-identical hormone replacement
therapy. I hoped her earlier hypothesis was right, connecting
my hormonal imbalance to the parasite. She urged me to rest
at home.

Within a few days, my waistline thickened, my body ached
and my head pounded. I finally shared the relapse with my best
friend, Rachel.

"Are you sure you don't have giardia? Your symptoms seem so
similar to last time."

I considered this possibility countless times. "Trust me, my
mother said the same thing but it's impossible. It's been too long
between showing any symptoms," I said, knowing the cysts take
up to six months to multiply, not two years. Rachel recommended the test regardless. I told her how much I dreaded seeing Jeff's
face when I announced the reopening of our giardia fund to pay

$395 for each test. I held off making an appointment with Dr. Cahill while I waited for the cortisol results.

After reviewing the latest blood work that showed a drop in my hormone levels, the doctor prescribed progesterone and testosterone creams at a pharmacy. She attributed the weight gain to fluid retention. It dawned on me that this was obvious, but I was so caught up in the minutia of gaining even one ounce that I missed the connection. I found myself in that dangerous place I swore I'd never go again—living my days based on the numbers of the scale. It terrified me how quickly any panic and frustration triggered these manic tendencies. When would it end?

I continued taking three supplements: Adrenavive, DHEA and Lodoral, to support my adrenal glands and thyroid until I received further information on the condition of my cortisol level. A few days later, the hormone creams arrived by messenger. That evening, I stood in my bathroom with Buddy laying at my feet and read the directions on the package. I wondered if I would blow up again like a balloon. I took a deep breath and looked down at Buddy. "Wish me luck," I said and began to apply the appropriate doses. I thoroughly rubbed each portion of the creams on the inside of my upper thighs and lower abdomen until it disappeared. I washed my hands and grabbed my black sweatpants off the ground, crumpled next to Buddy's face.

As I headed to bed, Buddy followed and lay on the floor next to me. He raised his eyebrows and lifted his head, tilting it as far back as possible, watching me get comfortable under the covers. While he rarely strayed from my side, I spent the majority of it repulsed around him. Even though I had chosen to keep Buddy for my family, I couldn't help but wonder if it was the wisest decision. I wanted to feel nothing but unconditional love for my dog. Instead, I had more resentment toward him as my condition worsened.

After ten days on the diet, I was actually heavier by only one pound than when I recovered from giardia in May 2011. The scale showed I was one pound from that healthy weight, but my body looked completely different. Clearly, the numbers didn't matter. I had been a prisoner to that scale and my whole obsession came to an abrupt end. At that very moment, I decided to toss my scale in the bathroom closet. I would no longer allow numbers to dictate my self-worth.

Even if I had lost weight on this crazy diet, I had stressed out my adrenal glands, causing my body to crash. There was nothing to celebrate. The victory I would have experienced, even momentarily, with the numbers on the scale, was and had always been an illusion. It was abnormal for anyone to drop weight this quickly. Who was I kidding? Coupled with a compromised immune system, I had only compounded the consequences.

The diet seemed harmless at the outset. I thought I made an informed decision based on the information I received. I assumed my body had built up enough strength and could resume most activities in moderation; however, in only eight months, my body reached its limit once again. What else did I need to know in order to understand that I could no longer live like this?

If I wanted to live a vibrant life, I had to make wiser and more permanent changes. I was like a serial monogamist, 'dating' one quick fix after another. I was obsessed about losing weight, not passionate about genuinely feeling good and creating any lasting wellbeing. Starved of self-love, I repeated the same sad story with the same sad ending.

My body was retaliating again with this second wake up call. I had to finally accept that even if my peers behaved in a similar manner, their genetic makeup and immune systems would create different results. Some might never show any signs of *dis*-ease. But my story was different. I had created every bit of this situation of unrest and ill health, and it was time to change the story once and for all.

When I woke the next morning, it took extra effort to open my eyes. I felt a searing sensation on the inside of my eyelids, hoping it was pink eye. I refused to believe the pain had anything to do with my past giardia symptoms. After Jeff had heard enough of my moaning, he offered to give the girls their breakfast before school, allowing me more time to rest. Once I got out of bed, I looked down at my distended abdomen, shocked to see the severe and aggressive bloat in my belly. Overnight, I had acquired a stomach as thick and round as a woman in her second trimester. I grabbed a sweatshirt to hide the obvious, then dragged myself to the bathroom to wash my face, hoping it would relieve the irritation in my eyes, which did nothing to make me feel better. I saw only a melancholic face looking back at me.

I was disappointed in myself that I once again let a doctor's point of view sway my decision to avoid all hormonal support. Clearly the excessive bloat had everything to do with the latest application of hormone creams.

When I finally made my way into the kitchen I kept quiet, sparing my family from further torment. I sounded like a broken record and had complained enough. I kissed Jeff and the girl's goodbye before they left for school. "Thanks for all the help this morning," I said, trying to cover up my sadness—and my grossly bloated belly.

"Just rest. I'll check in later," Jeff said.

I got up from the kitchen table and let Buddy inside after he tapped the sliding door. I bent down to wipe his paws and felt aches around the sides of my knee joints, reminiscent of past symptoms. I held onto a chair and pulled myself up, looking at

Buddy. "Boo, I have to go lie down for awhile," I said. He trotted ahead to the bedroom and plopped down on his pillows while I crawled into bed, ashamed by this harsh new reality: I had giardia again.

I rolled over, grabbed the telephone and called my mother.

"I understand it seems impossible but you should get tested anyway, just to be sure," she said. I considered her suggestion and, after hanging up, fell asleep within minutes.

Three hours later, I woke abruptly from the telephone ringing. I blinked several times, simultaneously glaring at the clock and reaching for the phone. It was Rachel. I decided to be honest and described my latest symptoms.

"I don't care what you say, I am convinced you have the parasite. You have to go regardless of the cost," she said. She was right.

I hung up and called the doctor's office, and scheduled an appointment two days later.

After dinner that night, my belly expanded even further, but now I felt pain and tightness that reached the top of my abdomen, recalling the days of beig hunched over in a ninety-degree angle. After Jeff put the girls to bed, I made my way to the den where he was watching television. I walked towards the couch, unzipping my sweatshirt to expose my skintight pink tanktop that was loose last summer. This was not the striptease my husband was hoping for. I turned sideways, keeping eye contact and waited for a reaction.

His eyes opened wide and his mouth fell open.

"You're kidding me. When did that happen?"

"It's been building throughout the day," I said, while Jeff sat quietly, staring at my belly. "I've got to have it, right? It's got to be giardia."

"How is that possible?" he asked, looking perplexed.

My vision became blurred with tears.

"I don't know, but I took those hormones last night and now look at me," I said, pointing my hands towards my stomach and continued, "My eyes burn, my joints ache and I feel like a walking zombie."

"What did the hormone doctor say?" he asked.

I sat down on the couch. "I set up a phone call with Dr. Galland for tomorrow and have an appointment with Dr. Cahill in two days. My mom and Rachel are convinced it's giardia. I'm having a hard time believing it myself but how else do you explain these symptoms and my reaction to the hormones? I have to rule it out."

Jeff turned away, facing the television and sighed while we sat in silence. Over the last four years, it was hard enough to keep up with the liability of my health condition from the first bout of giardia. We already scaled back on most of our expenses, hoping things turned around once I got healthy. Between that hardship and the decline in the economy, which greatly affected Jeff's business, we were barely treading water financially, and now emotionally.

It pained me that we had lost our connection, and that my husband was angry with me for something that originated with bringing a dog into our family. Deep down, I knew it wasn't my fault that I had giardia, yet I knew that the giardia was making me take responsibility for my behaviors that had contributed to the severity of my symptoms. It seemed like no matter what I told Jeff in regard to giardia, he could not believe the truth of its presence yet again in our lives. Often in those moments, I felt so alone, like a child with an angry parent, feeling powerless over what I could and could not do to help myself get through the pain.

He crossed his arms and shook his head. "We can't seem to get out from under our expenses and here we go again with the doctors."

My shoulders tightened and my cheeks stung from tears. "You think I want to deal with this all over again? Nine months ago I felt and looked great and now look at me." I knew our finances couldn't handle another round of medical attention.

I got up from the couch and walked out of the room then climbed into bed, turned on the television, feeling torn. If I had the parasite, I'd get antibiotics and heal faster, even if that meant more doctor bills, but if the results were negative, the expenses could be endless. I felt guilty that my family was about to face more debt. We had already cut back on most of our extra expenses.

Buddy pushed the bedroom door open with his nose and trotted across the room. He sat down next to my side of the bed and raised his paw for affection. He tilted his head back, hoping to get rubbed. Normally, I'd pull my hand out from under the covers and scratch his neck, but I glared at the tiny bubble-shaped saliva on his tongue. I hid my hands and blew him a kiss.

"Lie down Boo," I commanded, creating more space between us.

By the time Jeff came to bed, I was almost asleep. He kissed my head and said, "I'm sorry about before. The stress from everything is getting to me. I just can't believe a person's body can change that drastically in one day and if it's giardia, how the hell did you get it again?"

How the hell did I know, I wanted to scream. Instead, I said nothing, feeling the clutch of sadness and our eroding marriage. I shrugged my shoulders, and remained still, wondering if Jeff's giardia ever went away. It was hard to know because he never showed one symptom. Had I been re-infected by Buddy's saliva, sexual contact with Jeff, or unfiltered water from our faucets after the hurricane? I hoped both doctors had the answers.

Dr. Galland was equally surprised by how quickly my health had declined, reminding me of our conversation in October when I was well. I admitted my recent obsession with giardia research and writing my book, which resulted in a lack of sleep and exercise. I had also added some sensitive foods in my diet, stopped my probiotics and changed certain medications. I set up an appointment with Dr. Cahill the following day because the questions still haunted me.

He told me what I dreaded. It was possible to have been reinfected by giardia again. "It is also possible the infection was dormant inside your body and something activated it. Let's get the results from Dr. Cahill's test first and then we'll discuss options," he said.

Later that afternoon, when the girls came home from school and sat at the kitchen table doing homework, I blurted out my latest possibility. "I may have giardia again and have an appointment tomorrow to get tested," I said, hoping if I kept the girls in the loop it would make my fatigue and the situation more acceptable.

They simultaneously looked up from their papers as their mouths opened wide.

"Seriously, how do you know?" Jolie asked.

I stood up, unzipped my sweatshirt. "Because of this," I said and showed them my belly.

"Oh my God!" Abby said.

Jolie chimed in. "And you're the one who scrubs your hands all the time."

I sat back down.

"Do we have to take those pills again if you have it?" Jolie asked.

I understood her hesitancy, remembering the uncomfortable side effects from taking the first set of antibiotics. I reassured them we'd have more answers in the next couple of days.

"You're not thinking about getting rid of Buddy again, are you?" Jolie asked. Hearing his name, he came trotting toward her for a hug. She held him tightly and fixed her eyes on me.

I shook my head. "I don't plan on touching him until I know for sure," I said and looked the other way. I couldn't look in her eyes then. I kept my latest thoughts to myself for fear of devastating my family once again. After all this time, I assumed I was past any apprehension towards Buddy; however, the moment another infection was possible, I resorted to loving Buddy from afar. The irony struck me again—this time like an anvil. I loved Buddy but hated the giardia that came with him. Any sane person would have already gotten rid of their dog. Torn between the guilt of my family's reactions and the concern for my health, I had become the person I once resented: the people who looked at me aghast over my inability to see that this was making no sense. The dog was making me sick, period. Get rid of the dog: easy logic, hard to follow through.

I could not make this decision.

After dinner, the girls and I watched television in my bedroom. My mind drifted between the pros and cons of receiving a positive result within the next 24 hours. The anxiety made me curious about Adam's health. It had been a while since we connected and I hoped the parasite was long behind him. No one understood my headspace more than Adam.

I needed sympathy and reassurance and grabbed my cell phone to text him. *It's been awhile—I hope you're feeling better by now. Guess where I'll be tomorrow? Cahill's office—to get tested. Crazy right? I'll lyk my results!!!*

Adam answered immediately. *That's messed up!! I'm off antibiotics but still tired. Keep me posted. So crazy!!*

I read his message a couple times and harped on the word tired. It had been a month since he took antibiotics but he still felt fatigued. I did not know the details of Adam's reoccurrence, but I knew I was in for another long haul. This time, I was uncertain if I had the patience or stamina to endure more testing, waiting, medications, diets, supplements and the biggest uncertainty of all—how a new diagnosis would affect our finances and our marriage.

CHAPTER
22

I GAVE DR. CAHILL an accelerated version of the last nine months and finished by pulling the paper gown tight around my abdomen to emphasize the latest bloat. "Could it really be giardia?" I asked, trusting the country's most knowledgeable doctor on parasites to tell me the truth.

"Anything's possible. I take my patient's complaints into consideration, especially when they exhibit the same symptoms from the original infection," he said. Then he requested I lay down and turn on my side for a sample.

As he squeezed the jelly and prepared the scope, my body braced for the discomfort. I inundated him with questions, hoping to shift my attention. "It was over a year and a half before my symptoms first appeared so does that mean I was re-infected?"

"Let's see what your results show. If you test positive, then I would have the rest of your family checked, assuming one of them was the source of infection."

He reiterated how transmission occurs between husband and wife. When he left the room with the sample, I sat in silence, wondering about sexual contact with an asymptomatic person. Other than a quarterly scraping for $395, how could I trust that Jeff was clear of giardia? The stool test wasn't foolproof and there were enormous numbers of Americans still suffering—including me and possibly Jeff.

I peppered him with more questions. "Why did it take almost fourteen specialists to get an original diagnosis, especially now that I know constipation and bloat are symptoms of giardia? And if your test has proven better results, why is that not mandatory in hospitals and ERs? Shouldn't gastroenterologists use it at least? It doesn't make any sense. Over two million Americans get infected every year. That seems pretty prevalent to me."

He smiled, acknowledging that I had done my homework and read his book.

"Unfortunately, there are not enough studies done on this topic. It's not a money-maker like cancer," he said. He cited the ill effect of health insurance on the medical profession, and how gastro-enterologists give expensive procedures like colonoscopies and endoscopies instead because they get reimbursed.

I interrupted. "I know from personal experience that those two procedures don't diagnose giardia. If there was more awareness, wouldn't doctors recognize these symptoms and want to cut the statistics in half?"

"At some medical schools, there is only one day covered on the topic of parasites," Dr. Cahill said, having teaching experience.

"One day?" I asked, astounded. "How can that be?" It was no wonder that first emergency room doctor didn't connect my symptoms when I suggested, *My puppy has giardia. Do you think I could have it?* Like him, everyone else spent little time studying the parasite. How would these doctors know any better if medical schools barely broached this subject?

I didn't need to prove the doctors were wrong; I needed to reclaim my health and vitality. I had lived in survival mode for years, and I wanted to experience sustained wellbeing.

On my way out of his exam room, Dr. Cahill grabbed the eighth edition to his recently published book, *Tropical Medicine*. He signed the first page and handed me the book. "Read the introduction and epilogue. I think you'll find it helpful for your work," he said. As I headed to the front desk, he told me to call his office for my results after eleven o'clock the next day.

While I waited for my car in the parking garage, I opened the cover of the book and read his message: *For Tracey, As she finishes her first book—in good health. Best, Kevin Cahill.* I smiled, knowing whatever the test results proved, they were at least legitimate.

The hours before my diagnosis I had a sense of *déjà vu;* I sat in the same old spot on the den couch with Buddy close by, sporting the familiar pregnant-shaped belly. I spent enough time analyzing the probabilities and needed something else to pass the time before I made the anticipated call. I looked down at the coffee table and saw Dr. Cahill's book. I picked it up and began reading the suggested sections.

I was enthralled. Dr. Cahill recognized the importance for all physicians to have knowledge of clinical tropical medicine and to no longer restrict certain diseases by their geographic boundaries. He emphasized the need to view our world as part of a global community.

"The detection of tropical illnesses is utterly dependent on an awareness of their very existence, and on understanding their pathogenesis, signs, and symptoms," he wrote. "These fundamental facts are rarely taught in any depth in Western medical schools, and the diseases considered in this book—the greatest cripplersandkillersof theworld—rateonlypassingattentioninmost academic curricula in temperate climates."

I immediately flipped to the index and found giardia lamblia listed as one of the greatest cripplers. Other than the weight gain, my illness wasn't as obvious to the outsider, and no one—other than Adam—understood just how debilitating this infection was on the body.

I felt validated from Dr. Cahill's research and compelled to learn more. Apparently, giardia was not the focus of any medical research. Few American schools and hospitals taught the necessary disciplines, and therefore didn't attract the requisite funding for these kinds of infectious diseases. Further contributing to the rate of misdiagnosis were patterns of insurance payments. Even most of the doctors that Dr. Cahill trained over the years had turned to gastroenterology because certain procedures associated with the practice were reimbursed at higher levels than tropicalists.

Making matters worse, poor laboratory testing contributed to a lot of misdiagnosis. According to a 2010 study that checked specimens submitted to a major New York City university hospital laboratory—and one of the largest commercial medical laboratory in the area—"the hospital missed 50% and the commercial diagnostic inaccuracy was 70%." Apparently, Dr. Cahill's greatest frustrations were the same as mine. If enough attention was paid to these problems, I wondered how many giardia cases would get detected.

I glanced at the clock which read 11:02. I put down the book, picked up the phone and dialed Dr. Cahill's office.

The results were in: he found cysts in my stool sample, confirming the worst.

I had tested positive for giardia again.

More than two years after my first diagnosis, I made an ap-pointment for Jeff to be re-tested and a plan to submit Buddy's stool sample to his veterinarian. In the meanwhile, I waited for Dr. Galland's choice of antibiotics, wondering who was the source of my re-infection. I was definitely not touching Buddy or Jeff for a long time.

Dr. Galland recommended my whole family get tested this time. He prescribed two antibiotics to be taken together over the next nine days: 500 milligrams of Alinia and 200 milligrams of Albenza. I had to ingest two pills of each daily. He mentioned the various side effects I might experience but believed the large dosage was necessary to terminate the parasite.

I was less than thrilled that my girls had to undergo such an invasive scraping at ten and a half years old. Taking strong antibiotics wasn't the right option either since the medication could induce Colitis. I called Dr. Cahill's office, questioning the procedure on children, and was relieved to learn of an alternative to the scraping—the use of a finger instead. The girls would be anxious either way. No one wanted to deal with this again, but we had no choice.

I waited until Jeff got home from work and broke the news together during dinner. I cleared my throat and looked at the girls. "This time the doctor wants everyone to get tested, so I made an appointment for the both of you after the weekend."

Fear fell across both of their faces. The girls had overheard plenty of Jeff's jokes pertaining to the anal test. I continued.

"It's not done the same way as ours. There's no scraping.

It's only his finger."

"I guess that's better, but do we have to do the blood test?" Abby asked, professing her fear of needles.

"I don't care about that," Jolie said. "It's the other part that's annoying. I'd take the medicine over his finger." She nervously giggled, facing her sister.

"Trust me, I get it. Clearly nothing about this situation is going to be fun," I said, looking at Jeff. I saw approval, knowing I was seconds from a bribe. "If everything goes well at the doctor's office, then we can make a pit stop at Dylan's Candy Bar," I offered, turning their frowns into smiles.

The following morning, I reminded Jeff that we needed a fresh stool sample from Buddy.

"Seriously, you're telling me now?" he asked while I prepared the girls' breakfast as he was leaving for work.

I nodded and sat at the table. This was my second day on antibiotics and I already felt some effects: abdominal cramping, diarrhea and more fatigue. "Please, I am too tired to walk him and I refuse to wait another day for results," I mumbled. "Or touch him."

"You think he takes a crap on cue?" he asked, rolling his eyes.

I wanted to laugh but was too tired of this battle. I had nominated Jeff as the backyard collector of Buddy's stool. I only scooped during a neighborhood run, again double bagging and using gloves as if I was conducting a science experiment.

I wondered if Jeff recognized my recent detachment from Buddy. I had no problem talking to Buddy—that was easy—but I avoided responsibilities that exposed me to his germs: providing food, brushing his fur and teeth, cleaning whatever hair he shed on the floors, and even wiping his muddy paws on rainy days. If Jeff was suspicious of my behavior, he concealed it well.

Jeff sighed, grabbing Buddy's leash. "Hey Boo, apparently

mom says you need to go for a walk," he said, watching Buddy gallop towards the door.

"And don't come back without a sample," I teased, knowing this was Buddy's chance, once again, to prove his brilliance and devotion to us by crapping on cue.

Two days later, the veterinarian's office reported a clean stool sample. It was a relief to know Buddy wasn't the culprit this time, but I felt flustered, knowing it could be Jeff. It would have been easier to believe my dog infected me than my husband. I needed more reassurance from the veterinarian if I was to ever offer my unconditional love.

"I have a nurse who gets tapeworm from our patients just by looking at them even when she stands across the room," he chuckled, recognizing the number of people prone to certain infections. Was he kidding me? I knew that tapeworm was highly contagious but what did that mean? Would I ride the merry-go-round of giardia bouts forever? This parasite certainly wasn't a quick or cheap fix. I thought of more questions that would surface about my paranoia over my family's safety and my own.

I appreciated the veternarian's patience and extra time confirming the validity of an animal's stool sample. "If Buddy's results are negative, then he is definitely negative," he said, appeasing my ceaseless doubt. He offered further assistance if needed.

The discussion left me distraught. I still kept my distance from Buddy and spent more time in bed, believing it was the safest place in our house, but now the evidence pointed towards Jeff. Was our marital bed harming my health? Buddy's hairy wool pillows seemed more appealing than any connection with my husband. His appointment couldn't come fast enough.

The day finally arrived when the rest of my family got tested. The girls were scheduled at ten o'clock and Jeff at noon. Just before we got on the highway, I placed the Lidocaine cream on the inside creases of Abby's arms. "You swear it will be numb by the time he draws blood?" she asked, straightening her arms while I wrapped both areas within the plastic wrap.

"I promise," I said, exhausted. The medication had taken such a toll on my body that I wondered if it was also destroying the rest of me. My legs shook every time I stood up and the displeasing bathroom visits became more frequent. However, I pushed myself because the girls' tests were a priority, even if that meant we'd make an extra stop in the city to make up for it.

"Remember: don't touch anything," I reminded them when we walked into the doctor's office, ignoring their rolling eyes.

Once they entered the examination room and changed into gowns, the girls bickered over who went first. I sat in the extra seat with a lap full of clothes and no patience.

"It's fine. I'll go first," Jolie said. I smiled, assuming she knew I couldn't handle more.

When Dr. Cahill entered the room, he was friendly with the girls, explaining each procedure and made them feel as comfortable as possible. Twenty minutes later, he pulled off his gloves. "These samples aren't as accurate but I won't subject your children to the other test."

After the doctor left the room, the girls got dressed. I opened the door while they grabbed their coats and heard Abby say, "I have to go to the bathroom."

I groaned. "Really? Can you wait until we get to the parking garage?"

"Ugh, I really have to go. Why can't we just go here?"

The bathroom in a public parking garage seemed safer than a doctor's office that treated patients with the very diseases I feared.

I frowned. "Ab, we're in a parasitoligst's office, who sees patients for infections like mine. You might want to avoid the bathrooms."

Abby grunted while Jolie chimed in, "Mom, you're doing it again."

I chuckled. "Fine, but please triple-ply the seat with toilet paper and after you wash hands, don't touch anything else. Then I'll give you Purell."

We followed Abby into the bathroom and stood still while she went. I preferred to stand with shaky legs, watching my daughters' every move, than sit in the waiting room.

When Abby finished, I squirted Purell on both their hands, used a paper towel to turn the doorknob and angled my foot to help swing open the door. I tossed the towel in the garbage and walked down the hall, proud of my recent strategies to disinfect the bathroom.

Jolie said, "Hey Mom, maybe we should take a bath in Purell when we get home."

Everyone laughed, including me.

"I think you're on to something Jo," I said, pulling her in for a hug.

The next day while the girls were at school and Jeff was at work, it was hard to stay awake. Jeff set our bedroom alarm for ten o'clock so that I didn't miss the call from the doctor.

"Your husband and children are clean. Dr. Cahill found nothing," his secretary said.

I was dumbfounded by this news. "Are you sure you're looking at my husband's file?"

"I guess you were expecting different results," she said, suggesting I follow up with Dr. Galland. I hung up the phone and called Jeff with the news.

"I knew it wasn't me," he hollered, questioning why I wasn't sharing in his joy.

Though I was relieved that everyone was clean, then what was still making me sick? I rolled onto my side and stared at Buddy, a constant reminder of the original source of infection. The only option left to consider was that the parasite never left my body and waited for the right environment to thrive.

CHAPTER
23

O N April Fool's Day, I tossed the last two antibiotics in my mouth and washed them down with bottled water. The day of jokes was not lost on me. Had I played a huge part in recreating this mess or was it all just a coincidence?

I hoped the first round of heavy-duty medications would help. I spent a lot of time in bed, sleeping hours at a time or simply lying half comatose, imagining critters crawling inside my body. I was eager for a follow-up scraping, but had to wait two weeks before Dr. Cahill's retest. The only thing that left me a little more at ease was knowing that I would meet Dr. Galland in two days.

The moment I entered his office, I spewed my concerns. "If my whole family tested negative for the parasite, where does that leave me?"

"Let's test the water in your house just to be safe," he said, peering over the rim of his eyeglasses. "Since no one else in your household is infected, it seems the parasite was, in fact, dormant."

He reiterated how stress weakens the immune system, causing activation, and he reviewed which actions caused the most strain on my body. Nothing he said seemed surprising after our phone call the previous October. He continued to connect the dots.

"Giardia can feed off gluten."

I sat back and paused for a moment. "Really? I didn't realize that," I said, wondering how I missed such an important component. Although my food allergen tests proved high gluten intolerance, my symptoms were never life-threatening enough that I had to carry an EpiPen in case I went into anaphylactic shock. For several years, I did my best to avoid the sensitive foods on my list, especially gluten, but I assumed the worst-case scenario resulted in some bloat, constipation, fatigue or even weight gain. In the past, I believed wheat products were a healthier choice.

I never looked at gluten as hazardous to my health until now. Though I had not read *Wheat Belly* at the time, my understanding of gluten had changed after learning how these products affected blood sugar levels more than any other carbohydrate. According to *Wheat Belly*, gluten causes high glucose and provokes visceral fat accumulation, causing the muscles and liver to respond less to insulin. In order to metabolize the sugars, the pancreas has to make large quantities of insulin. At that point, the body gets stuck in a vicious circle of insulin resistance, insulin production, and deposition of visceral fat, producing inflammation in the body's cells—and creating a "wheat belly" among other harmful conditions.

Dr. Galland explained that the bloat related to eating wheat is probably due to fermentation in the gut. If one has Celiac Disease or a wheat allergy, the bloat may be directly associated with inflammation. If sensitivity to wheat causes bloating, it's because humans poorly digest the glutinous starch in the wheat. An overgrowth of bacteria or other organisms in the small intestines contributes to the fermentation of that starch, which produces the bloat. It was clear these actions had a domino effect and created a place for the parasite to thrive. Without probiotics, I stripped my gut of any good bacteria. I ate the foods that gave the parasite strength and behaved in ways that placed additional strain on my body. It was obvious how serious I needed to be about making informed decisions and permanent changes in regard to my diet.

Dr. Galland ordered a prescription of Vitamin B12 injections, hoping my energy levels increased while he waited for the results of Dr. Cahill's retest, reminding me that I needed a negative result before he could proceed.

"I'll see you in a month. Feel better," he said.

I was confident that the source of infection wasn't coming from contaminated water, but I continued to use bottled water even while I brushed my teeth. I waited until I had enough stamina to take on the doctor's suggestion to check my household's water supply. Then I dove in and researched water system companies, read their yearly reports, and called related organizations for further explanations of test requirements and findings.

A week later, some of my fatigue had lifted. I wasn't sure if it was the antibiotics or the Vitamin B12 shots that helped, but it didn't matter. I was thrilled to be out of bed, resuming most of my daily responsibilities around the house. I took Buddy on short walks in the neighborhood, completed basic errands for my family, attended the girls' lacrosse games and even kept our Saturday night plans—a miracle considering how long it had been since I got off the couch. When my body needed rest, I listened and napped in the late afternoons or went to bed earlier, making the healing process a top priority.

This newfound energy came at the perfect time and motivated me to answer questions about the water. After I finished a morning walk with Buddy, I went online and searched my township's water department and dialed the number. I was transferred to several different divisions and spoke with a handful of people, asking basic questions. Does the town water get tested for giardia? What's the difference between well water and surface water? Are there state guidelines that mandate testing for giardia specifically?

According to the 2011 New Jersey American Water report, roughly thirty samples were taken each month, both tested primarily for two types of bacteria, E. coli-a bacterium and coliform which cause acute sickness. When traces of bacteria existed, the water was treated and samples were retested until cleared. I was aware of the difference between bacteria and microorganisms and asked about protozoas.

The top two microorganisms, cryptosporidium and giardia, have both caused acute waterborne illnesses in the United States. It was only when new data on cryptosporidium proved to have acute cases during a Minnesota outbreak that it received more attention and concern in the press, especially since acute giardiasis had already existed for a long time. I was told that in 2003 the Environmental Protection Agency had proposed the Long Term 2 Enhanced Surface Water Treatment Rule. I looked online and found the regulation which stipulated treatments for 14,000 water systems, including surface water and ground water used by 180 million people. The findings provided only two years of monthly sampling for cryptosporidium. To reduce costs, small filtered water systems monitored E. coli-a bacterium. The pathogen cryptosporidium would be monitored only if E. coli exceeded specified concentration levels, which led me back to my original question. Was anyone specifically testing our country's water for giardia?

After much run around at New Jersey American Water, The Environmental Protection Agency and New Jersey Department of Health, it seemed that the only reason giardia may get sampled is because it occurs at times with cryptosporidium. It was also explained that when found in samples, the water would then be disinfected with additives like chlorine to inactivate the pathogens. This process was supposed to reassure me that our water systems were clean. I was told this information by the same person who thought giardia cysts could only live outside the human body for a few days at best, which was incorrect. I wanted to show them my belly.

I inquired about getting the tap water in my house sampled but was told I needed to hire a company certified in testing giardia. Apparently, there are only three laboratories in the United States that are certified, none of which are in New Jersey. After being told that a private home test could cost roughly $1,200, I avoided another financial meltdown with Jeff. At this point, my brain was fried from an overload of information. I tossed the research aside and made sure I had an adequate supply of bottled water, trusting Dr. Galland's theory that the parasite was dormant.

I was eager to progress with my recovery, which meant another scraping. While I dressed for my appointment, Abby came in the bedroom complaining of a bellyache. I felt her forehead and took her temperature, which seemed normal. "You're probably just tired and should get to sleep earlier tonight," I said, suggesting she get dressed for school. Buddy remained on his pillows with one eye opened, watching me. As I left the bedroom, he got up and followed.

I walked past Abby's room and found her resting in bed. "I really don't feel good, Mom," she said, begging to stay home.

Buddy lay by my feet while I sat with Abby in silence. I was torn, knowing Abby didn't skip school unless she truly wasn't feeling well, but this appointment was also too important for me to miss. I let her rest and talked it over with Jeff, who wasn't able to stay home with her either. When I came back to Abby's room, Buddy was still in the same spot.

"Can I just go to your appointment and sleep when we get home?" Abby asked.

I agreed, knowing my past appointments were rather quick.

After I fed Buddy, I took a box of melba toast on our way out in case she got hungry at some point during the trip to New York City. Thirty minutes into driving on the highway, I heard her retching.

"Mom," she said.

I looked in the rearview mirror. Oh shit, I thought, tearing open the box of melba toast and tossing the unopened bags on the floor. "Use the box, Ab. Use the box," I said, hoping she could open it wide enough and miss the upholstery and rug. Thank god she had good aim.

Once we got out of the Lincoln Tunnel and stopped at the first traffic light, I turned around, hoping to provide some comfort. She was sound asleep and used the seatbelt to prop her head up while never losing grip of the box between her legs. We pulled into the parking garage, a block and a half away from the doctor's office. I took the ticket from the parking attendant and opened Abby's door, placing the box on the backseat floor. I caressed her cheek.

"We're here honey."

It took a few seconds for Abby to open her eyes. She was pale and barely moved. "Can you carry me, please?" she asked. It was only three years ago, but everything about this mirrored the time Abby had the swine flu: I was sick with the same condition and heard my daughter's whimpering for help, while standing in a parking lot before a doctor's appointment.

I took a deep breath, lifted her body and headed up the ramp, holding what felt like dead weight. As we approached the street corner, her soft voice whispered in my ear. "I'm going to be sick again, I need to get down," she said, gently swaying her feet.

I looked for an immediate solution, regretting that I had left the melba toast box in the car. "We're almost there," I said and suggested she wait for the closest bathroom—inside the doctor's office.

"I can't make it," she said. I worried she'd vomit on herself or a pedestrian as they walked past us. I looked around one last time, spotting a public garbage pail—our only option—and hurried over, praying she would make it.

"Here," I said, setting her down in front of the pail and pulling back her hair. "Just lean over it and try not to touch anything"

She turned her head and faced my direction. "Eww, I can't," she said as tears filled her eyes. She paused for another minute. "It's only another block, right? I'll try to make it to the doctor's office," she said, raising her arms up, signaling she wanted to cross the street. We made it halfway through the next block before we sat down on the sidewalk where my daughter vomited. She glanced at me from the corner of her eye, apologizing that she couldn't wait.

When she was finished, I lifted her up, walking like a person fleeing the crime scene. Her head softly bounced on my shoulder. "What about my throw up?"

It never crossed my mind in Abby's condition she'd even care about the mess.

"I don't have anything to clean it," I said.

"But we can't just leave it there. Isn't that considered littering?"

My eyes bulged. Who was the responsible adult now?

"I'm sure it'll rain in the next day anyway," I said, praying that I was right.

She gently sighed in my ear but reluctantly went with me to the doctor's office. I cleaned her face in the bathroom, careful not to touch anything but the paper towels, then took my test twenty minutes later. Abby was silent until I got dressed. She hadn't said much the whole time, and I knew she was still thinking about the mess on the sidewalk.

"Of all people, you don't have wipes in your bag?" she asked, leaving us both laughing.

Five days later, I got out of bed on a Sunday morning and opened the window, breathing the fresh air of a perfect spring day, reveling in my clean bill of health from Dr. Cahill. I was free of giardia. While some of the lethargy faded, the rest of my symptoms remained. At least I had the foresight to know my recovery would take time. I pressed my cheek against the screen and closed my eyes, listening to the chirping birds and smelling freshly cut grass and cherry trees in bloom.

I dressed in gym clothes, tied the laces to my sneakers and grabbed the iPod, no longer solely motivated by weight loss. I simply wanted to feel the connection with the earth.

When I entered the kitchen, Jeff looked up and smiled.

"It's nice to see you heading outside," he said.

I grinned, putting my ear buds in place. "I'll probably only be fifteen minutes," I said, aware of the stamina I needed to rebuild again. "It's such a gorgeous day. When I get back, we should take everyone to the school park."

Jeff agreed and hollered for the girls to get dressed and collect their lacrosse sticks. "I'm assuming you haven't fed Buddy?" he asked, barely smiling.

I headed outside, brushing off his comment and stood in the driveway, listening to music and stretching my legs. I took a deep breath, honoring the gift of being outside. I headed down the block, grateful to see the beauty of the crisp green grass and my neighbors' colorful landscapes. Four songs later, my legs got tired and I stopped and turned around.

While I walked up the last hill, I looked down at the street sewer to my right, where three years ago, I had collapsed. This was the place where Buddy and I reconnected while racing each other home after our morning walks in the neighborhood. I recognized it now as a place of forgiveness and acceptance, and, for the first time, felt peace and gratitude for all I had survived.

I was eager to spend the rest of the afternoon with my family. When I returned, everyone was in the garage and ready to leave for the park. Jolie grabbed her bicycle while Abby chose a scooter. Jeff held onto Buddy's leash and I took the girls' lacrosse sticks as we walked down the hill. "Girls, stay close to the sidewalk," Jeff shouted, watching as they raced past us. Buddy tried to follow suit but Jeff yanked on his leash to slow him down. "Don't worry Boo, you'll get your chance to run once we get to the field," he said. I glanced to my left, acknowledging the sewer I passed only moments before and shared my latest insights with Jeff.

He wrapped his arm around my shoulder and held me tight. "Trace, it's really nice to see you less focused on the trivial things and rising above it all this time. I know it sucks that your symptoms are back, but hopefully it won't take as long to heal," he said and kissed my forehead.

Despite Jeff's pride, my family's smiling faces and my personal growth, I still wasn't sure if I was rising above my feelings towards Buddy. I loved him but he brought giardia into my life which had been both a curse and a blessing. I avoided sharing these thoughts with anyone. Clearly, I was apprehensive. Every time I touched him, giardia came to mind. Even though I knew he wasn't the reason I got sick this time, I was tormented by possibilities. But, this wasn't the time to worry about what may come. I mentally regrouped and focused on having fun with my family.

The girls waited for us on the field. Wearing gloves for protection, I took Buddy's leash from Jeff and handed him their lacrosse sticks. While they practiced lacrosse drills, I took Buddy to the basketball courts and kneeled, petting his head. He sat still. His eyes were solely fixated on me. I knew he wanted his own playtime, which meant he wanted to run free. I shouted in Jeff's direction. "You think he'll be fine if I let go of the leash?"

"Definitely, let him go," Jeff said with confidence.

Jolie dropped her lacrosse stick and ran over to join us.

I smiled, seeing Buddy looking back at me. "Aw, Boo," I said, wishing he could understand my actions and appreciation for the unconditional love he had given me. I dropped his leash.

"Go, Boo. Run free," I said, hoping he'd run for me.

Buddy galloped off into the beaming sunlight. I wrapped my arm around Jolie and watched Buddy run huge circles across the field, while his fur blew in the breeze. My smile widened, feeling like a proud parent. He sprinted with an opened mouth. I wasn't sure if I'd ever have the kind of stamina to run like him or even with him, but it didn't matter. Watching him run filled me with a new and profound pleasure, and I decided then that life without Buddy would not be possible. I would just have to remain vigilant.

Jolie grabbed my iPhone and took pictures. Abby stopped playing and came over to us. When Buddy turned and darted towards the other end of the field, Jolie looked at me.

"Mom, what if he keeps running in the other direction?"

I chuckled, thinking about the times I was faced with Buddy's game of chase. "Sweetie, he's not going anywhere when his family is right here. He'll come back, trust me," I said.

"Worst case, we can always get some Trader Joe's chicken,"

Abby said with a huge smile. I laughed and she continued, "Or a Bijon Frisee that I want!"

Abby repetitively shared her desire for a second dog, empha-sizing the need for a small one. I even pictured Buddy carrying this new best friend in his mouth around the house, until I saw myself wearing gloves and a facemask. There was no way I would indulge this fantasy.

Buddy stopped by Jeff's feet, looking to play fetch. Jeff grabbed a tennis ball and tossed it in the field. As the ball arced across the grass, Buddy dug up the dirt with his paws. Then he ran off, search-ing for the ball and gave up. I looked at Jeff and laughed when Buddy trotted back to us. "You might not be the best retriever, but you are certainly golden," I said, watching Jolie bend down and hug him, wishing that one day, I could love him just as freely.

CHAPTER
24

Fueled by accepting my current health and body size, I was feeling better by the spring of 2012, even though my symptoms had not completely disappeared. By May, Dr. Galland prescribed a familiar protocol with Fluconazole and Clotrimazole lozenges to treat yeast overgrowth. He gave me probiotics, digestive enzymes and natural supplements to support my adrenal glands and stimulate brain function. I left his office confident that my recovery time would be shortened; however, over the next two weeks, the fatigue slowly crept back.

My bright world was fading quickly.

I immediately made an appointment with my acupuncturist. After all the time I had spent in Chris's office, I gained an exorbitant amount of scientific knowledge, a trust in holistic medicine and a friendship. It was well worth my time and resources to seek his help again.

"Do you know how many of my patients come back to me, wondering why they've relapsed and then proceed to tell me they added gluten back into their diet, knowing they have an allergy to it?" he asked, reiterating the havoc food sensitivities have in one's body. I explained my need for variety and that I felt deprived from the lack of food choices. He flicked me a look with raised brows. He didn't have to lecture me. I knew no matter what my reasons were for stopping the probiotics and adding back the foods, it was irrelevant now.

Even though I was feeling healthier, my adrenal glands and reserves needed more time to be replenished. Chris wasn't going to let me get away with anything. While he inserted the needles, he asked, "The HCG diet, really?"

I felt foolish and didn't say anything, laid on my back, bracing for the lecture that I needed to hear again. "That is something you just can't mess around with. It definitely puts additional strain on the body," he said, wishing I had thought to discuss it with him first.

"Trust me, I get it now," I said without any sarcasm. Chris was totally right.

"It would be great if everyone saw their setbacks as opportunities to change their behaviors," he said, turning off the lights on his way out of the room. I closed my eyes, listening to a visualization meditation on my iPod and recommitted to seeing him twice a week.

I had another round of inflammation before my second acupuncture treatment, two days before my forty-first birthday. With the fatigue creeping back, all I cared about was resting. Instead of going out for my birthday, friends brought over their kids, sushi and cake to celebrate at home. While the kids made a mess of our basement, we hung out in the den enjoying each other's company. Within an hour of dinner, my stomach was cramped and bloated. I tried to stay silent, figuring my friends had heard enough complaints from the aftermath of giardia, but I got too uncomfortable. "I have to change into sweatpants," I said, busting out of my jeans.

When I came back, I lifted my shirt and turned sideways, displaying the size of my belly to my close friend Wendy. Her mouth opened wide. "Oh my God! When did that happen? Because it wasn't like that when we got here," she said, baffled by the quick progression.

"It just happened," I said, feeling like I had just pulled off the greatest magic trick—one David Blaine could never replicate. My belly went from looking like it was at the beginning of a pregnancy to expanding within an hour into a third trimester ball. I had only eaten a few pieces of sashimi fish and one cup of plain brown rice and was as perplexed as everyone else as to how this could happen. Unlike a true magician, I didn't have the capability to return to normal.

Since there was nothing to do but wait and wonder, I continued to stay present for our company. When it came time to blow out the candles on the cake, my wish was obvious.

The next morning when I woke up, I was extremely exhausted and bloated. The more exhausted I felt, the more bloated I became, making it clear these two symptoms went hand in hand. I even had Jolie take some pictures from the various angles, texting my parents and Wendy with a caption, *the morning after—can you believe?* While friends witnessed the abnormal size of my belly over the years, no one other than my family watched it actually expand in the blink of an eye. It didn't matter how many times I was told it was a result of food sensitivities and inflammation in my gut, a hormonal reaction from the parasite, or even food malabsorption, I was still dumbfounded and now utterly devastated that the end was nowhere in sight.

I called Dr. Galland first thing Monday morning and shared my latest setback, assuming the cysts had multiplied again. He suggested I set up another retest. Two days later, I underwent another scraping and received a call from Dr. Cahill. While he didn't find cysts on my lining walls, he found traces of Charcot-Leydan crystals. This was a new term for me.

Apparently, the crystals are not produced by giardia. The immune response to the parasite may produce these crystals. They are the result of the activation of a particular type of immune cell; they're the smoke rather than the fire. Given my history and current symptoms, Dr. Cahill's recommendation to Dr. Galland was to treat me with a different antibiotic and for a longer period, hoping to clean out my insides once and for all.

Dr. Galland prescribed 250 milligrams of Paromomycin Sulfate capsules. I was to take two pills, three times daily over the next ten days and received a warning about abdominal cramping and more fatigue. Although I was a pro at handling these hardcore antibiotics, I dreaded the consequences of consuming sixty pills in less than two weeks.

The first evening on the medicine, I attended a temple service for my girls' Hebrew school class. They wore silky spring blouses and cute skirts, while I stood in my bedroom and tried on four different dressy shirts, hoping I could cover the bloated belly without buttoning my black slacks. I squeezed into a pair of Spanx tights and put on a smile for the girls.

Once we got to temple, I sat down and rested my head against Jeff's shoulder, avoided socializing with anyone and hoped I'd stay awake through the service. On our way out, we bumped into

Adam and his wife. Other than a few health updates through text, we had not corresponded. At this point, he was clean and trying to heal. I tried to sound positive but a few complaints crept into our conversation.

When Jeff walked over, Adam asked if I knew of a certain holistic doctor that was recommended to him. I motioned to Jeff with little energy. "That's the mad scientist guy," I said, insisting he run the other direction but desperately wishing someone had the solution.

For the ten days I took the mega dose of antibiotics, I slept while the girls were at school. I had two weekend bar mitzvahs in a row and needed as much time to recover as possible. It felt as if someone had injected me with multiple doses of morphine, leaving me unconscious for hours, drooling on my pillow. When I was awake, I was grateful that I could move at all. On one of the last nights of this treatment, I felt Jeff climb under the covers but had no energy to snuggle or offer any touch at all. I couldn't handle it any more.

I stared at Buddy while Jeff set the alarm clock. "I hate that I'm completely paranoid around him," I said and told him the story about the vet's nurse. "I'm terrified, Jeff. I can't live here like this anymore." I turned toward the wall because I couldn't bear to see his face. "Either we get rid of the dog or I have to leave this household."

He grabbed my arm and leaned over my shoulder. "Trace, listen to me. After everything you've been through, I get it," he said, wiping my cheeks, "If we have to give him up, then that's what we have to do. Eventually, the girls will understand," he said, kissing my forehead. The last thing I wanted to do was to shatter my girls' world.

Three weeks later, I had my third follow-up visit with Dr. Galland and felt tremendous relief. This time, the fogginess had vanished, the fatigue had lifted and the bloat had quickly subsided. I was finally free of the parasite. The antibiotics had brought me back to life. Other than the extra eighteen pounds I carried, my condition seemed easier to handle the second time around. Dr. Galland gave me a new prescription, cutting my thyroid medication in half to 90 milligrams. He questioned if I needed to stay at such a high dosage anymore. I stopped questioning anything at this point, even if this was just another false summit in the long journey.

It was the last week in June. I now had seven weeks to focus on weight loss with the girls at summer camp. I could hardly believe they had just graduated from elementary school. It seemed like yesterday when Jolie jumped off the kindergarten steps, landing in my arms, bursting with enthusiasm over the latest series of books she found in the media center—*The Tales of Biscuit the Puppy*. Her teacher had shouted, "Mrs. Berkowitz, someone has a new love and has been talking about it all day."

That was the first time Jolie had mentioned her desire for a dog, prompting my own illusion of what comprised the perfect life. On her last day of fifth grade, she flew out those same school doors, filled with her very own puppy tales. Only this version was far from the fantasy any of us imagined.

CHAPTER
25

THAT SUMMER, I still battled with extra weight, but I refused to give up. By mid-July, Dr. Galland offered a prescription of Cycloset. When he mentioned it was another form of Bromocryptine, my mind drifted, wondering why the name sounded familiar. He said that Cycloset was used by Diabetes Type 2 patients because it helped lower blood sugar.

"I took this medication once before," I said, recalling a month of negative side effects. He flipped through my thick file and reviewed the dosage, leaving the decision to me.

I sat for a moment, taking into consideration that my health was in much better condition and decided it was worth another shot.

After eight weeks on Cycloset with nausea and fatigue, I discontinued the medication. Even though I dropped five pounds, the side effects weren't worth it. My priority was my health and eating healthy. My spirit was revived and in better condition than ever to deal with this. I researched different websites for more gentle ways to heal my body, reading updated posts from other giardiasis sufferers who used natural supplements to maintain their health. When I found MSM, a nutritional form of biological sulfur known to prevent giardia, my curiosity piqued.

I consulted Chris and he recommended adding certain herbal supplements to my current regimen. I took GI-Synergy, which combined three capsules in one package: Yeastonil, which dealt with yeast and fungus overgrowth, Parastonil, which managed parasite problems for anyone diagnosed with intestinal parasites or high blood IgE levels, and H-PLR, which supported the immune system during minor bacterial, fungal and parasitic infections.

I understood the importance of optimal intestinal health and knew it was necessary if I wanted my endocrine, neurological and immune systems to function properly. When I ran out of Dr. Galland's probiotic, I switched to Strengthia and also added Repairvite to restore and maintain a healthy intestinal tract. He also gave me Adaptocrine for my adrenal glands, which reduced the effects of stress on my body, and AdrenaCalm, a cream that aids in balancing the cortisol levels in the bloodstream.

After my latest relapse, I knew I had to see my body as a whole system. Every weak link hindered another system. If the adrenal glands struggled, imbalances were bound to coexist based on my genetic makeup. I also knew that years of negative behaviors placed a strain or even blocked the cellular communication of the very feedback loop Chris discussed, which contributed to my *dis*-ease when the relay of information broke down.

My chronic health condition had been effected by "power outages," where cell sites were down for months at a time, even years, and missed their connections because of blocked outlets. It was hard to believe I was as ignorant about the causes of my own illness as most of my doctors. My condition was spelled out for me numerous times and yet, I traded obsessions like baseball cards, never acknowledging the series of behavioral patterns and false beliefs that actually damaged my body, mind and spirit. It was then that I knew I had to find a healthier way to release negative emotions brought on by these daily stressors.

Eventually, I found helpful, healthy tools. I listened to meditations, inspirational speakers, and uplifting music on my iPod during morning walks or short distance runs with Buddy, in the car or before bed, sometimes for as little as ten minutes per day. They all helped to bring some sense of calm. The more I welcomed these routines, the more I felt a positive shift in my energy and experienced moments of ease. The results provided a better relationship between my body, mind and spirit, and I was willing to let my guard down around Buddy. My paranoia hadn't completely vanished, though: I diligently washed my hands after every hug, but my affection for Buddy became more consistent. When he nudged my hand for affection with the tip of his nose, I stopped pulling away. I even caught myself mindlessly petting his fur, without any revulsion. I no longer felt disgusted seeing his fur on my clothes and on the floors. We could have a future.

Things were starting to align for me. People and opportunities were showing up to reflect what I needed to learn. I never considered the root of all these synchronicities. The closest I ever came to understanding 'spirituality' was reading the book, *The Middle Place* by Kelly Corrigan. Her story about being a mother of two young girls while dealing with her own illness amazed me. She rose above her own circumstances and shared her lessons with others.

It was no coincidence that the subject of energy medicine appeared and how it related to one's balance of health. I absorbed as much information as I could. After reading *Anatomy of Spirit* by Caroline Myss and *Body of Health* by Dr. Francesca McCartney, it was clear that illness went hand in hand with one's psychological and emotional issues, beliefs and attitudes. Both books demonstrated different tools and skills to develop and reach a state of wellness.

Acupuncture was at the top of my list to cleanse my body of emotional stress. When I started treatments it was with a vague understanding of how these so-called blockages got rerouted, but I felt better after every session and became a believer in the benefits of acupuncture. Ancient Chinese call the life energy coursing through our bodies *Qi* and say it is stimulated by needles on the surface of one's body through meridians of acupuncture points which redirects the flow of life energy. Once the communication gets re-routed, our bodies get stronger and heal.

My weekly treatments left me at ease. Every time I entered Chris's office, I was excited to absorb the next scientific topic of the day. I finished each session by listening to the tranquil sounds and voices from different meditations on my iPod. After years of hardcore gym workouts, which I had hoped would release such tensions, I am now able to lay back and follow the rhythmic pace of my breath to achieve peace of mind while keeping my moderate exercise routine intact.

Every time I walked up Chris's stone path to his office, I silenced my cell phone and smiled, embracing the serenity. By the end of the August, my vitality was finally rejuvenated. At social functions, I was no longer concerned about what I would wear or how people perceived me. I wanted to hear how other people were doing instead of telling them about myself.

I was ready to leap back into life—this time with a profoundly different perspective. I wanted to participate with my whole being, not some half-baked idea of who I was based on what I

looked like or the façade of what our society created, but on how
I felt and how I responded to adversity. I was feeling gratitude
every day and my body was coming alive again. It was literally
time to test the waters.

When the girls returned from camp, we went to a friend's lake
house in the Berkshires for a short vacation while Buddy spent
time with other dogs at our groomer's store. I shoved the extra
bags of bottled supplements, medications, foods and blender in
the trunk, content with my routine; however, when we unloaded,
I noticed the perplexed look on our friend Peter's face.

"What is all that stuff?" he asked.

"This is what's getting me healthy," I said with confidence.

"And making me broke," Jeff added, providing a laugh for
everyone.

Jen and I made all the beds and got the kids situated. By the
time my head hit the pillow, I was exhausted but eager to wake
the next morning and smell the fresh country air. I loved everything about the lake house, except the lake.

Sunlight shined through the window as I quietly got out of
bed. I couldn't get my gym clothes and sneakers on fast enough
for a short run around the lake. After I took my necessary medications, Vitamin B12 injection and supplements, I left the house
and headed down the wooded path, blasting my iPod, longing
for my companion, knowing how much Buddy would appreciate
the new smells and sights.

A few hundred feet up on the right was an opening to one of
the large grassy, tree-filled fields that gave way to the lake. I was
in awe of the stillness of the water and slowed down. Something
about this place filled me with a sense of calm. I sat down at the
base of a birch tree and faced the lake, breathing deeply while
I listened to my playlist. I smiled, looking out at that beautiful
lake, imagining Buddy by my side. The serene atmosphere was

extremely seductive, yet I couldn't forget that this was a place I also feared. Amidst all that beauty was the lurking monster in the lake—the possibility of giardia. There must have been millions of parasites in that water, and I knew at some point my daughters were going to ask me to swim.

Unsurprisingly, the girls popped the question two days later, even though they were not the biggest fans of lake water either. The dads left Sunday evening, needing to be at work early Monday morning. I decided to curb my fears and joined them that afternoon.

"All right, I'm going in. Who's coming with me?" I asked, surprising even myself.

The girls' mouths opened in shock, and I smiled. They knew this was a huge moment for all of us. I sprinted toward the dock so that I could not change my mind, though my heart pounded and I felt butterflies deep in my stomach.

Jolie hopped into a kayak while Abby stood waiting for me.

"Are you ready Mom?" she asked, reaching her arm out to grab hold of my hand.

I blew her a kiss, appreciating the warmth from our entwined fingers.

The closer I got to the edge of the dock, the more I regretted the decision. I even considered running for cover but refused to let my paranoia keep me from participating in this moment, or anything in life. It was too late. I needed to do this, not just for myself, but also for my girls. I found myself internally repeating *"I can do this"* and *"Stay in the moment."* We got to the edge of the dock, glanced at each other one last time and I took a deep breath.

"I'm ready," I proclaimed.

Abby counted to three. I pinched my nose and squeezed my lips as tightly as possible. We bent our knees and jumped, plunging into the water. We let go of each other's hands and I kicked with all my strength to get my face above the surface. Something happened in that moment between the descent into those dark waters and the second I saw light again. I'm not a believer in baptism, but this was clearly a rebirth. I would never in a million years have believed I would plunge into a lake, just to have fun, despite the infinite threats to my health. The only thing that mattered to me was the ability to connect with a profound and primal joy, a right I had denied myself for so long, that I wanted to weep in those waters—not for everything the giardia had taken from me, but for what I had denied myself for most of my life. Submerged in the lake, I spread my fingers in the water and reclaimed my right to optimal health and joyful living.

I broke the surface and gasped for air, then wiped my eyes. Abby flashed me a smile while Jolie paddled over in her kayak, applauding my efforts. We swam another twenty feet and climbed onto the floating dock. I sat next to Abby and watched Jolie bobbing around us, feeling the buzz of joy but wondered how long I'd have to recover until Abby was ready to swim again.

The paranoia crept back immediately. By the time I reached the dock and got out of the water, I grabbed my towel and dreamed of being hosed down in Purell. I would have gladly ingested a full prescription of antibiotics, too.

A few hours later, when Jolie finished her shower, she joined me in the bedroom and got dressed. "I can't believe you went into the lake today. Why did you?" she asked.

I grinned. "Because you girls wanted me to," I said, putting on my tanktop. "Although I'll probably have giardia again and look like the Good Year Blimp in about a month."

"Mom, you're too funny," she said and laughed.

Despite all the germaphobic paranoia and health concerns, I had to live my life, regardless of my fears. I was determined to find beauty in the outdoors and keep a sense of humor about it. I wanted my girls to know that despite the many challenges life throws at us, we have a choice in how we respond to them. I may never look like I wanted to again, but I know I could learn to love my new life. After all of this, I wanted to offer that ultimate lesson to my girls.

The next morning, we packed the rest of our belongings and spent time tidying the house before we headed home. Between the many late nights, glasses of wine and constant fun, my throat was sore when I swallowed. When Jen and I finally climbed into her car with the kids, I could barely reach over my right shoulder to grab the seatbelt. My eyes and head ached. I leaned against the seat, realizing this was just another sign that my immune system was still vulnerable.

Jen looked over at me. "Are you okay, Trace?"

I took a deep breath, certain that I was getting sick. "Not really, but I'll be fine," I sighed, putting a smile on my face. Halfway through our ride, my throat flared up even more as if a golf ball had lodged itself there. My body continued to weaken with fatigue.

I looked at Jen. "Can you believe how sick I am already?" I said, noticing how quickly this crept up on me. When we got home, I crawled into bed, petting Buddy's head. I barely left the bedroom for the rest of the week. I was wise enough now to listen to my body when it screamed it needed to rest.

By September 2012, it was time to see another endocrinologist who specialized in Integrative Medicine. My weight was at a standstill and I had this strange feeling that something else was being overlooked after I got strep throat during my long weekend at the lake house.

I should not have been feeling as crummy as I was given my good spirits only a few weeks prior. The fluctuations in temperament were as frustrating as the lingering weight, though I wasn't as concerned about what I looked like now. I worried about how I felt. I could only fake a smile for so long.

I needed a doctor to request blood work. I consulted with Chris about the right person, keeping my expenses in mind. He shared the name of a woman in New York that his other patients recommended.

"Apparently, she suggests a lot of supplements. You just have to be careful."

I knew enough about supplements that I could refuse anything that would waste my time and money. A few weeks later, I pulled my thick portfolio from the kitchen drawer and brought it to my appointment. The doctor spoke with a heavy German accent. She listened to a summary of my journey while skimming through the applicable paperwork, occasionally circling certain results. She mumbled, "Yep, uh huh," compelling me to take a peek.

She looked up, flipping her pencil between her fingers and asked, "Wow. Did anyone ever mention your high acid levels?"

I was silent for a moment. "Yes, at one point in my recovery I took natural supplements to help lower those levels," I said, realizing that information came from the mad scientist.

She explained that people can only stay healthy if the body has a balance between its levels of acid and alkaline or as she referred to it, "optimal pH balance." Apparently, the fluids, blood and tissues in a body must remain alkaline in order to be in good health. She explained that acid is created in our bodies by digestion and the production of our own energy, and that the body is always working to maintain this balance. When a person's pH levels become too acidic from toxins and stress, mineral depletion, or an acidic diet, the body becomes susceptible to a variety of health issues. She flipped through the rest of my blood results.

"Your acid levels remained consistently high through the years. No wonder you got sick again," she said.

I stared at her, perplexed, wondering if the mad scientist had actually spoken some truth.

She handed me a pen and sheet of paper to write down my new protocol. In the morning, on an empty stomach, I was to take a probiotic with Chlorella in water in order to detoxify my body. I understood this basic process completely. She suggested I buy a juicer and juice twice a day using dark leafy greens, avocado, lemon, sprouts, and measured amounts of coconut and primrose oils. Those directions were simple enough to follow and the rest of my diet would stay the same.

Then she spewed off a number of new supplements that I couldn't write down fast enough. The paper was filled with scribbles in my rush to jot down every word. She recommended I buy a water ionizer for our household, claiming I would shed the remainder of the weight once my body was more alkaline. At the same time, she also mentioned I purchase an Alkapod, a to-go container for the car that uses minerals to balance the alkaline levels in unfiltered water. This was the most important suggestion and could be a solution to my fear of drinking water in public places. She turned to her computer screen and scrolled down the list of choices, making reference to the more expensive ones. All I saw were dollar signs—two thousand to be exact. I knew there was validity to achieving pH balance but I was over-whelmed with the additional costs. If I felt this way, how the hell was Jeff going to handle it? We both hoped this was the last medical advice.

The doctor took more than fourteen vials of blood. "My first-time patients are usually panicked by these drastic changes," she said. "You seem to be only half panicked since you have some experience." She smiled, pulling off the rubber band from my arm.

Had I shown up in her office two years ago, I might have left confused and in tears, but I knew better by then and needed time to process everything. I made a follow-up appointment for the next month, giving these new products enough time to take effect.

Jeff called on the way home. "How did the appointment go?"

"My head's spinning, but I think good," I said, determined to research every product.

I started juicing immediately, which left me more energized each morning through lunch. I purchased some of the suggested supplements and skipped a few others. I researched all different brands of water ionizers and called a few companies, settling on one that was reasonably priced. I even sent Jeff a few different links, explaining the importance of an alkaline balanced body in order to keep healthy and vibrant, including how diet soda lowers one's pH balance dramatically, which convinced Jeff to eliminate most soda from his own diet.

By the time I had my next appointment, I dropped another five pounds and was eager to hear the results of my latest blood work. The doctor handed me roughly nine pages of results. As she reviewed each one, I wrote down more suggested supplements. I flipped through the pages and noticed a sheet of food allergies. I squinted, scanning the paper. A moment later, I looked up and asked, "You tested me for food allergies?"

She nodded. "I've seen people hold onto weight because they are eating foods they're allergic to," she said. She pulled out her copy of those results.

I looked to the left side of the sheet where it listed the range of severity.

"Most of the foods have the number two beside it and the rest have the number one. Do I have to avoid all twenty-five?" I asked.

"For now, cut all those foods in order to clean out your system. Unfortunately, the foods that have a number two listed next to them will need to be permanent," she said.

When I turned the page, I read a list of different inhalants in the environment, which didn't seem to be an issue. The test proved uncertainty with specific trees, pollen, dust and penicillium, but my mouth dropped open when I reached the bottom of the list.

"No way," I said, looking directly in the doctor's eyes. "There's a number one next to dogs and cats."

She nodded. My mind ran in a million directions. Was this the moment of truth? Would she tell me I had to get rid of Buddy once and for all, even though I had finally let go of past doubts? I braced for the answer feeling a cold sweat.

"It's positive but on the lower side. That means you may get cold-like symptoms as a reaction from his hair," she said.

I took a breath and stared at the paperwork. I could deal with a cold. I could cough, I could sneeze, I could expel the stickiest of phlegm balls. Bring it on, I thought. What I could never do is end the relationship that had started all of this, my choice to bring that ball of fur and boundless love into our family on Memorial Day weekend years ago.

Buddy had experienced the ups and downs of my condition just as much as Jeff and the girls. While they had indulged him with enormous affection and treats, I had left him alone and ignored him for stretches of time during my sickness. Neither of us could get that time back. It was gone and all I had left was a choice about how I would move forward with Buddy in our lives, learning that it wasn't just the giardia, but his fur that had made me ill all this time.

For almost five years, Buddy had seen a magnitude of sunrises and sunsets, traveled through numerous grassy fields and treasured the smells of the fresh outdoors with us. Not unlike most other dogs, he had also been left behind, watching his family shuffling in and out of our house as we lived our lives. He never once retaliated or withdrew from us, but waited patiently to hear one of us call his name. "Buddy, come here!" Every time my throat itched or nose sniffled, I would be reminded of the unconditional love he gave us. Buddy deserved the same devotion in return.

I stared again at the test results, feeling resolved. Even if Buddy's presence caused me to hold onto excess weight, his presence in my life was permanent.

"So we'll vacuum the house more often. I'll deal!" I shouted.

The doctor looked at me strangely, struck by my wild enthusiasm. She had no idea what had just transpired for me and spent the last ten minutes discussing the benefits of using power magnets, which act as a natural antibiotic on the body. She suggested I buy one of the company's products, specifically a mattress pad in order to get the full effects at night. This was another expensive product that sounded enticing but I needed to investigate it further.

When I left her office, the only thing on my mind was the list of food allergies. While I had fully accepted the consequences of keeping Buddy in our life, I struggled to accept the elimination of gluten, soy, dairy and peanuts from my diet. During brief moments when I felt food deprived, my immediate symptoms were reminder enough to surrender to this song and dance. Now the forbidden food list included apples, almonds, white beans, beef, chicken, corn, eggs, garlic, pork, potatoes, oranges, shellfish, tomatoes, tuna and all rice. By this point, I already knew how my immune system over- compensated for the inflammation those foods caused. I immediately changed my diet, since I had already eliminated these same foods for eight months after an allergen test indicated my sensitivities in 2010. I wasn't partially allergic. Only a fool would indulge in eating these foods again until my digestive system healed—which could very well take a few more years.

When I showed the list to Chris at my next acupuncture treatment, he agreed with this latest protocol, confident that my body would soon start shedding the excess weight. I shared my latest meal plan, still somewhat dismayed by the limited choices: a vegetable juice for breakfast, either plain grilled salmon or turkey burger with a salad for lunch and the opposite protein with quinoa and sautéed vegetables at dinner. I snacked on one serving of walnuts, pistachios or sunflower seeds in case I was hungry. No doubt, I'd lose weight with this plan.

"Why don't you put some salmon in the juicer in the morning?" he asked, making light of my situation.

"Great idea," I said, smiling, appreciating his acknowledgement of my commitment to get healthy.

Over the next few weeks, I contemplated the purchase of $1,000 king size mattress pad full of power magnets. I was seduced by the idea of extra healing while I slept, assuming it would expedite my recovery. After I called the company and inquired about a twin mattress pad, I had the opposite opinion. I learned that this magical mattress pad was only a few inches thick, and it was possible that a person who slept on the other half of the bed would experience "long term effects" such as burn marks on their arms and legs because they got too close to the sides of the 'magnetic' mattress. Seriously. It was all I needed to know.

I laughed when I shared this latest clarification with Jeff.

"So the negative magnets drip towards the sides of the mattress pad and may burn my arms but the positive magnetic field stays on top for healing?" he asked, trying to keep a straight face. "What if you roll over and your own arm falls off to the side? Or worse, what if something else happens to flop over and hit the force field?"

We howled over this concept and the threats to precious anatomy.

"I'm glad you find this ridiculous as well," he said.

I appreciated that Jeff finally acknowledged the change in me, seeing the joy in my face and knowing that I could still laugh no matter what came next on this wild ride with my health. We were trying to find our way back to each other day by day. Our marriage struggled, and we recognized that. I refused to live behind a façade of perfection anymore. I had no idea how any of this would end; the stark truth was that we had drifted apart. It was all very unsettling in its clarity.

I wasn't desperate for quick fixes and was able to stand up for myself when something didn't feel right. I decided the limits of supplements and what I put inside my body. I might never get back into my size 2 clothes but that didn't scare me anymore.

I had faith that my body would settle at a healthy size, not what the fashion magazines dictated. I had Buddy and a whole new appreciation and respect for what was in my power to control and change—and ultimately accepted the circumstances that needed to change me.

Slowly, I was finding more contentment despite the small tests that continued to enter my life. When flu season struck in January 2013, the girls came home from school in a panic. Jolie ran to the kitchen table where I was working and dropped her school bag on the floor, petting Buddy while rambling about a conversation she had with her sixth grade English teacher.

"I told her I was thirsty and asked to get my water bottle in my locker," she said, bypassing her teacher's suggestion to use the water fountain down the hall.

After everything we had been through with my condition, we both knew she would rather stay thirsty than drink from a water fountain. Apparently, Jolie's expression of disgust was a reflection of my own.

"Oh my god, Jolie, what did you tell her?" I asked, laughing at our craziness.

"I just said it was because of germs," she said, giggling while kissing Buddy's face.

"The flu is going around in case she didn't understand," I said, wondering what exactly she had told her teacher. I imagined the glazed-over look that most people gave me. *A parasite can do all that?* It didn't matter if the teacher understood or what anybody else thought. I was one person against an army, speaking the truth. A parasite had brought me to my knees.

Though swimming in lakes would never become a habit for me or a form of exercise, I knew I had to find another way to move my body. Clearly, running long distance wasn't an option any more and, after everything I learned, I had made peace with that. However, I needed another activity that would align with my new body.

I had always loved to dance and wondered if I could muster up the courage to step back into a dance class. My sister first introduced me to Niyolates when we moved into the suburbs—in 1998. That was fifteen years ago, but the memory was fresh.

Huge mirrors covered the walls. Oh no, I thought. We can *see* our-selves? I wasn't sure about this situation. The lights dimmed as a hint of daylight filtered through the front window. Twenty barefoot women of all ages dressed in sports bras, gym tanktops and exercise pants moved about the hardwood floors with an ease that astonished me.

Rolin, the male instructor, announced each movement through a microphone headset. The women flawlessly swayed their hips, achieved repetitive squats or balanced during leg lifts. As if these moves weren't impressive enough, they effortlessly shimmied their shoulders and skillfully expanded their fingers and arms to the beat of Latin, Hip-Hop, Pop, Rap, Motown and other sensual music.

Who knew what double front and back leads were? I kept tripping over my own feet as I listened to the instructor's directions, "Double diagonal, back cross, side, center and change."

I watched the other women with envy. Why couldn't I move like them? I felt like a big clod and wanted to run out the door. While the dancers focused on improving their mind-body connection through breath, I was fixated on looking like a bumbling idiot and missed the bigger picture. I couldn't shut my mind off for one hour, let go of my body image and just have fun. But this wasn't fun. Far from it. I couldn't escape noticing my lack of coordination, flexibility and balance—and I was convinced everyone else noticed too in those huge mirrors.

In that moment, it didn't matter that I ran miles every day. Watching their movements reminded me that I didn't have the finesse the other women seemed to easily possess. I tried to turn my attention to the music and listen to it instead of the gremlins in my head.

I appreciated the diversity of music and the "good" kind of soreness my body felt days later. I noticed aches I never had after running and weight training. Once the class ended, I told my sister, "I'm clearly not cut out for this, but I can tell why you like it. It's too bad I can't dance like them."

She chuckled and waved her hand.

"It takes everyone a few classes to get the hang of it. You should try it again."

I don't think so, I thought. I couldn't commit to another class too soon. I was still too self-critical to know this form of movement was exactly what my body needed then.

Fifteen years later, a friend who taught a spin class at a studio twenty minutes from our neighborhood mentioned Rolin when describing other classes offered there.

My mouth opened. "I took a Niyolates class by an instructor with the same name years ago! It's got to be the same guy," I said, wondering if I should try it again.

Synchronicity was clearly guiding our conversation. It had been years since I heard anything about this class and now learned Rolin owned a studio which focused on mind-body connection.

I searched on my cell phone for his website. *"Pursue kindness, wellness and peace of mind. The rest will follow."* After everything I learned from my journey, I had the foresight to be open-minded now, concentrating on the importance of how our bodies respond to the way we think, feel and act.

The following week, I drove to the Bodies-inMotion Wellness Studio and tried the class again. Mirrors covered only the front wall of the new space. I stoodon the glossy wood floors, which reminded me of the last class many years ago. While I stared at my reflection, Rolin greeted me. We shook hands and got reacquainted with each other as I reminded him of the class I tried years ago.

As the music started, Rolin uttered directions into the microphone. There were the double front and back leads, tightening our abdominals as we shook our hips, shoulders, arms and fingers to flush out the lymphatic system. We did grapevines, squat downs, leg lifts and shuffled our feet sideways, front, center and back while we focused on our posture alignments.

Rolin repeated, "Smile, relax your facial expression. Let your body go."

I assumed he directed those comments towards me. I consistently stumbled and felt tense. I found myself frustrated once again. Halfway through the class, the woman besides me leaned over and whispered, "It takes a few classes to know what you're doing. Just keep coming. We've all been there."

Immediately, my shoulders loosened and I relaxed the rest of class even though I couldn't get the steps right. Just before class ended, Rolin said, "When you control breath, you control movement. Breathe in the future, exhale the past."

I connected with the music and his words that morning and was hooked on the class. The woman who stood next to me that first day was right. It took a few classes to catch onto the movements but I'm learning daily how to free my mind and let my self go—without overexerting my body through long distance running.

Nowadays, when the alarm clock sounds, Buddy lays on his pillows with one eye open, watching my every move. He stares as I dress in gym clothes, preparing for his morning walk before I leave for dance class. His tail wags and he stays still until I reach for my sneakers. At six years old, Buddy knows the routine, even if that means he waits until I return from dropping the girls off at middle school. He still accompanies me all the way to the garage door, regardless of my plans with him. Holding the doorknob, I watch as my daughters place their emptied plates into the dishwasher before gathering their belongings and even witness as

Jolie offers Abby her lunch bag because she had forgotten it in the fridge. I glance over their chosen outfits and freshly blown hair. I take it all in, admiring their individualized style while recalling how much of their childhood was experienced in my absence. After years of agonizing over the effects of my illness, it's moments like these I see how much they have flourished into independent and compassionate people.

When the girls and I are ready to leave the house, they kiss Buddy one last time.

"I promise I'll be back for you soon, Boo," I say, closing the door behind me.

As I drive back up the street, I see his face in our front window, waiting for my return. He watches while I pull into the driveway then disappears. I know he's racing to the doorway for a greeting. Whichever direction I go, he follows and waits.

After a few minutes alone in the bathroom, I hear something tap on the door. I push it open and see him, head tilted sideways, staring at me with a quizzical expression. I am still floored by his manners, knowing he has never scratched for anybody else or on anything other than the sliding door in our kitchen.

"Don't worry, Boo. I'm almost done," I say.

When I get close enough to the cabinet where I keep his leash, he gallops to the door, smacking his tail against the wall from excitement, making it difficult to hold back my laughter.

"Guess you're ready today, huh?" I ask and attach the leash to his collar. I shove two empty bags into my windbreaker pocket, set my iPod to a playlist, slide on gloves and close the garage door. As I stretch on the driveway and look at the sky, Buddy takes in the scents. I can't help but grin, acknowledging our mutual love for the great outdoors. My priority isn't about running miles with my golden boy anymore. I solely focus on the companionship and adventures we share. Nothing is off limits anymore.

His fur, muddy paws and gentle touch remind me that I can love him freely now. Buddy helped me find contentment within myself and that is the greatest gift of all.

The End

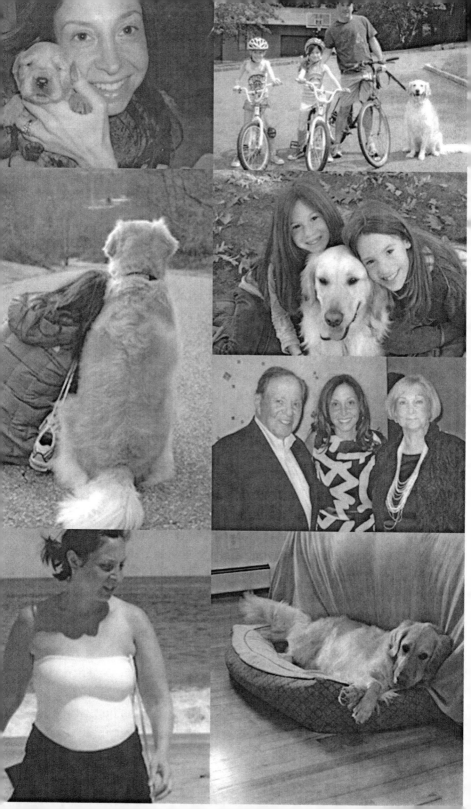

ACKNOWLEDGEMENTS

FIRST AND FOREMOST, I feel extremely fortunate to have met and collaborated with my writing coach, editor and friend, Holly Lynn Payne. Your guidance, love for the craft and insight helped bring my story to life. Thank you for introducing me to some of the most talented people who contributed to the birth of *Not My Buddy*. Tom Joyce, your creativity, design work and patience is immeasurable. Joaquin Lowe, I am grateful for your honesty and sharp editorial suggestions in the final draft. Jayme Johnson, your vision and attention to detail helped turn my ideas into an amazing platform. Melanie Sazegar, your assurance in my story and ingenuity for marketing helped target my audience.

Thank you to my medical team: Dr. Daniel Zacharias, Christopher Butler, Dr. Margaret Nachtigall, Susan Horowitz, Dr. Philip Felig and Kathleen D'Agati, who gave everything they had to help me recover. Thank you, Dr. Leo Galland and Dr. Kevin Cahill, for your time and patience guiding me through my recovery and for providing pertinent scientific information for the book and website. Rolin San Juan and Susan Richter, you have been a huge part of my self-growth. I am eager to pass on the knowledge to those still suffering and, hopefully, raise awareness in our country.

To my parents, Judy and Fred, your encouragement and support over the years have been endless. Mom, you truly are my tower of strength. Your dedication and unconditional love for our family has taught me how to persevere through all of life's challenges. Dad, thank you for the foresight and belief that my story will make a difference in other people's lives. There is no greater compliment than witnessing a father boasting over his children's work. Apparently, I learned something from my four years at Ohio State other than partying. To my amazing sister Melissa Trachtman, you are my first friend and second mother.

Kelly Corrigan, your wisdom and inspiration portrayed in *The Middle Place* gave me the faith that I too, a stay-at-home mother, can write a book. Thank you for offering suggestions in your acknowledgements page. I took your advice and fortunately found more than one 'Phoebe' who insisted I kept writing. Jennifer Cohen, Rachel Stern, Nicole Dersovitz and Marni Statmore, thank you for the encouragement.

Thank you to my family, friends and early readers for your invaluable direction, additions and honest critiques: Gail Rosen, Alix Trachtman, Wendy Lenchner, Adam Karp, Cathy Levison, Lori and Samantha Alpert, Nancy and Michael Wolk, Scott Stern, Adam Gittlin, Louise Vyent, Leslie Lavinthal Sandy Patschke, Norma Ketchersid, Trudy Quinn, Lisa Kent, Andrea Fine, and Justin Spencer.

And finally, Jeff, it's been quite a journey. Your patience and understanding throughout the years are gifts I will always cherish. We are extremely blessed to have brought our beautiful daughters, Abby and Jolie into the world. Girls, you are the sole reason I strive to be a better mother and more compassionate person. The way you handled yourselves during my sickness was extraordinary. You amaze me every day. It's because of you that Buddy entered our lives and made me who I am today. Thank God we didn't pick the runt!

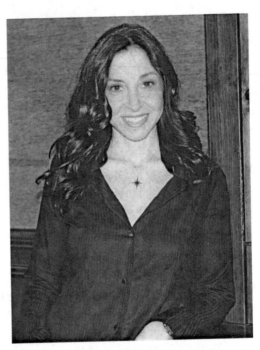

TRACEY BERKOWITZ is an advocate for people suffering from chronic giardiasis. She lives in Livingston, New Jersey with her twin daughters and dog, Buddy. She received her BA from Ohio State University and worked as a part-time preschool teacher. *Not My Buddy* is her first book.

---

www.traceyberkowitz.com
Facebook: Author/Tracey Berkowitz
    Group/A Chronic Giardiasis Community
Twitter: @t_berkowitz
Instagram: t_berkowitz
www.pinterest.com/traceyberkowitz
https://www.goodreads.com/author/show/
    12596263.Tracey_Berkowitz

CPSIA information can be obtained at www.ICGtesting.com
Printed in the USA
LVOW10s1951080616

491762LV00023B/1262/P